The International Behavioural

MENTAL HEALTH AND
CONTEMPORARY THOUGHT

TAVISTOCK

The International Behavioural and Social Sciences Library

MENTAL HEALTH
In 8 Volumes

MENTAL HEALTH AND CONTEMPORARY THOUGHT

Volume Two of a Report
of an International and
Interprofessional Study Group
convened by the World
Federation for Mental Health

EDITED BY KENNETH SODDY
AND ROBERT H AHRENFELDT,
WITH THE ASSISTANCE OF
MARY C KIDSON

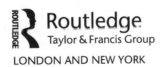

LONDON AND NEW YORK

First published in 1967 by
Tavistock Publications Limited

Published in 2001 by
Routledge
2 Park Square, Milton Park, Abingdon, Oxfordshire OX14 4RN
711 Third Avenue, New York, NY 10017

First issued in paperback 2014

Routledge is an imprint of the Taylor and Francis Group, an informa business

© 1967 Kenneth Soddy

The publishers have made every effort to contact authors/copyright holders
of the works reprinted in the *International Behavioural and Social Sciences
Library*. This has not been possible in every case, however, and we would
welcome correspondence from those individuals/companies we have been
unable to trace.

These reprints are taken from original copies of each book. In many cases
the condition of these originals is not perfect. The publisher has gone to
great lengths to ensure the quality of these reprints, but wishes to point
out that certain characteristics of the original copies will, of necessity, be
apparent in reprints thereof.

British Library Cataloguing in Publication Data
A CIP catalogue record for this book
is available from the British Library

Mental Health and Contemporary Thought
ISBN 0-415-26455-3
Mental Health: 8 Volumes
ISBN 0-415-26511-8
The International Behavioural and Social Sciences Library
112 Volumes
ISBN 0-415-25670-4

ISBN 13: 978-1-138-86745-1 (pbk)
ISBN 13: 978-0-415-26455-6 (hbk)

Mental Health and Contemporary Thought

Volume II of a Report of an International and Interprofessional Study Group convened by the World Federation for Mental Health

Edited by KENNETH SODDY
and ROBERT H. AHRENFELDT
with the assistance of Mary C. Kidson

TAVISTOCK PUBLICATIONS

J. B. LIPPINCOTT COMPANY

© *Kenneth Soddy, 1967*

First published in 1967
by Tavistock Publications Limited
2 Park Square, Milton Park, Abingdon, Oxon, OX14 4RN
in 11 pt Plantin
by Butler & Tanner Ltd, Frome and London
Distributed in the United States of America and Canada
by J. B. Lippincott Company, Philadelphia and Montreal

To
JOHN RAWLINGS REES, C.B.E., M.D., F.R.C.P.,
this report in three volumes is affectionately
dedicated by the members of the
International Study Group
on Mental Health Perspectives, 1961

Volume I Mental Health in a Changing World
Volume II Mental Health and Contemporary Thought
Volume III Mental Health in the Service of the Community

Contents

CONTENTS

Acknowledgements

Grateful acknowledgement is made to the National Institute of Mental Health, US Public Health Service, for US PHS Research Grant No. M-4998, which made it possible for the International Study Group to meet, for the summary report *Mental Health in International Perspective* to be prepared, and for editorial work on the current report in three volumes to be started; to the Grant Foundation of New York for bearing the cost of the salaries of the members of the Scientific Division of WFMH; to the Council for International Organizations of Medical Sciences for a subvention towards the preparation of resource materials; and to the WFMH US Committee Inc. for a grant towards the completion of the bibliography included in these volumes.

Thanks are due to Faber & Faber Limited, London, and Oxford University Press, Inc., New York, for permission to quote from his *Collected Poems, 1925–1948* the poem 'Prognosis' by Louis MacNeice, which appears on pages 245–6 of this volume.

Obituary

ALBERT DEUTSCH died, suddenly and peacefully, in his sleep on Sunday, 18 June 1961, the seventh day in the work programme of the Study Group with which this Report is concerned. He was an experienced science writer and journalist, and perhaps the most distinguished 'communicator' in the field of mental health. His main assignment with the Study Group, in which he also took an active part, was to write the summary report for presentation at the International Congress on Mental Health in Paris, August–September 1961.

For thirty years Albert Deutsch had been completely dedicated to the task of raising the level of understanding in the United States of the problems of mental ill health, and made immense contributions to the promotion of awareness both of the need for change and of means towards its achievement.

Participants

The participants in the International Study Group came from eleven countries and represented fifteen fields of professional work. Their names, and their professional appointments at the time of the Study Group, are listed below:

DR H. C. RÜMKE (*Chairman*)
Professor of Psychiatry, University of Utrecht; Member, Royal Academy of Sciences in the Netherlands

DR ROBERT H. AHRENFELDT
Psychiatrist; Consultant and Research Associate, WFMH; *formerly* Dep. Asst Director of Army Psychiatry, War Office (UK)

THE REV. GEORGE C. ANDERSON
Director, Academy of Religion and Mental Health, New York

DR SIMON BIESHEUVEL
Director, National Institute for Personnel Research, South African Council for Scientific and Industrial Research, Johannesburg

†MR ALBERT DEUTSCH
Editor-in-Chief, *Encyclopaedia of Mental Health*, Washington, D.C.

DR JACK R. EWALT
Professor of Psychiatry, Harvard University Medical School; Superintendent, Massachusetts Mental Health Center; Director, Joint Commission on Mental Illness and Health, USA

DR RICHARD H. FOX
Psychiatrist, Bethlem Royal and Maudsley Hospitals; Hon. Asst Secretary, Research Committee, Mental Health Research Fund, UK; Secretary, Medical Research Council (UK) Sub-committee on Psychopathic Personality

DR FRANK FREMONT-SMITH
Director, Interdisciplinary Conference Program, American Institute of Biological Sciences; President and Chairman, Governing Board, WFMH US Committee Inc.; Co-Chairman, World Mental Health Year Committee

DR OTTO KLINEBERG
Professor and Chairman, Department of Social Psychology, Columbia University

DR DAVID M. LEVY
Lecturer in Psychiatry, College of Physicians and Surgeons, Columbia University; Consulting Psychiatrist, New York City Dept of Health; Visiting Professor of Psychiatry, Tulane University Medical School, New Orleans

DR TSUNG-YI LIN
Professor of Psychiatry, National Taiwan University Medical College, Taipei, Taiwan

DR STEPHEN A. MACKEITH
Consultant Psychiatrist and Physician Superintendent, Warlingham Park Hospital, Surrey; Adviser in Psychiatry to the County Borough of Croydon, Surrey; Consultant Psychiatrist, Mayday Hospital, Croydon   .

DR MARGARET MEAD
Visiting Professor of Anthropology, Menninger School of Psychiatry; Associate Curator of Ethnology, American Museum of Natural History; Adjunct Professor of Anthropology, Columbia University; Visiting Professor of Anthropology, School of Psychiatry, College of Medicine, University of Cincinnati

DR BEN S. MORRIS
Professor of Education and Director of the Institute of Education, University of Bristol

DR A. C. PACHECO E SILVA
Professor of Clinical Psychiatry, Faculty of Medicine, University of São Paulo, and School of Medicine of São Paulo; President, WFMH, 1960–61

DR JOHN R. REES
Director, WFMH

DR AASE G. SKARD
  Associate Professor, Department of Child Psychology, University of Oslo

DR KENNETH SODDY
  Scientific Director, WFMH; Physician and Lecturer in Child Psychiatry, University College Hospital and Medical School, London

DR GEORGE S. STEVENSON
  Editor, *Mental Hygiene* (NAMH quarterly); President, WFMH, 1961–62; *formerly* National and International Consultant, NAMH; Medical Director, National Committee for Mental Hygiene, USA

DR ALAN STOLLER
  Chief Clinical Officer, Mental Hygiene Authority, State of Victoria, Australia

DR MOTTRAM P. TORRE
  Assistant Director, WFMH; Asst Attending Psychiatrist, St Luke's Hospital, New York

DR CLAUDE VEIL
  Psychiatre de l'Association Interprofessionnelle des Centres Médicaux du Travail, Paris; Chargé de Conférences Techniques à l'Institut de Psychologie, Paris; Secrétaire du Groupe d'Hygiène Mentale Industrielle (Ligue d'Hygiène Mentale)

WHO Observers:
†DR E. EDUARDO KRAPF
  Chief, Mental Health Section, WHO (*died 9 December 1963*)

DR DONALD F. BUCKLE
  Regional Officer for Mental Health, WHO, Regional Office for Europe

DR TIGANI EL MAHI
  Regional Adviser for Mental Health, WHO, Regional Office for the Eastern Mediterranean

Preface

It is with great pleasure that I have accepted the invitation to write a preface for the Report in three volumes of the International Study Group convened by the World Federation for Mental Health in 1961. For me, as Chairman of the Study Group, the reading of the manuscript has revived many memories of this fascinating meeting and stimulated a great number of thoughts. I believe that the Report is of the greatest importance not only for those of us who had the good fortune to be members of the Study Group, but also for all those who are interested in both the scientific basis and the practice of mental health. In these restless and changing days, with their unending series of unpredictable international tensions, it may reasonably be asked whether it was worth while for a small group of men and women of widely varying individual scientific interests to come together in remote and lovely surroundings merely for the purpose of talking with each other. Although they had prepared working papers for the meeting and a number of references to the literature had been collected, they came without prepared scientific papers, 'official' documents, important statistical findings, films, or other concrete evidence, and also without an agreed conceptual foundation for the meeting. What they did bring with them was their experience of many and various forms of psychiatry, clinical and social psychology, sociology, education, or religion.

Within a prepared framework, which was designed more or less to cover the field of mental health, the Study Group spent its time in extempore discussion ranging over the oldest, the newest, and the most urgent problems of human beings. The conceptual aim of the conference was to provide an open exchange of thoughts, experiences, and views among a group of people of wide and varied experience, and by so doing to make a contribution to the science of man by the integration of the most diverse and highly specialized personal experience. The long-term hope was that the resulting synthesis of experience might make the sciences of man of greater value in the endeavour to improve mental health all over the world.

It is sometimes asked whether it is possible to achieve such ends by merely talking, and whether the not inconsiderable sums of money involved are well spent. Many of those who have been brought up in the natural science disciplines are not in sympathy with this type of programme. Natural scientists today are preoccupied with their attempts to raise the levels of methodological precision, to reach a higher level of objectivity, to clarify their models of thought, and to advance new hypotheses in the search for scientific principles. We can perfectly understand the point of view that the aims of the natural scientist as defined cannot be furthered by group discussion. On the other hand, we hope that many natural scientists are aware of the more intangible factors that appear to be operating in the field of the human mind and of the relationships between people, and that they may be willing to agree that the special conditions obtaining in the field of mental health may require alternative and additional methods of approach.

We would ask the natural science purist who is unable to make any concession to a less pragmatic method of operation not to concern himself overmuch with these volumes. The purist is not likely to find a great deal of value in this Report. He will be distressed by a comparative lack of objectivity, and his scientific self-confidence may lead him into the detection of many errors. Above all, he will be greatly concerned by the lack of scientific proof for much that occupied the International Study Group's time.

Those who took part in the Study Group are fully convinced that such heterogeneous interprofessional and transcultural discussions are of high potential value, provided they are properly prepared and imaginatively planned. It is our conviction that this way of working enables us to arrive at the sources of new thinking. The work in which we are engaged in advancing the scientific knowledge of mental health is still only at its very beginning. The phase in which we are now working may fairly be called 'pre-scientific' – a necessary precursor of more objectively scientific ways of working. In our view, it is premature to narrow our interests to an exclusive specialization and search for objectivity. There is a place for both kinds of work – more concern with objectivity is urgently needed, but at the same time we need to preserve a view of the whole field in order to see more clearly the relative values of the many lines of specialized inquiry.

In this 'pre-scientific' era of mental health work, the primary need is to know how best to relate the many and various findings over the whole range of the field, at a time when much of the practical work that is being carried on is not of a highly specialized order. Major advances in conceptualization are not possible without the cooperation of a multidisciplined team. It has been said with some truth that from multidisciplined to undisciplined thinking is only one step. But, on the other hand, multidisciplinary thinking is the best defence against both the overestimation and the underestimation of the results of single-disciplined work. Only the multidisciplinary approach is likely to lead us to whole and basic truths.

This Report gives a number of perspectives over the whole of human life. Its subject-matter, which ranges widely around the world, will enrich the reader. The great complexity of the material and the diversity of thought may well have a confusing effect, but throughout the Report the connecting factor is the human being – Man as he is today in an ever-changing environment. If the reader is able to keep this connecting thread always in his mind, he will be at the same time surprised at the wide variety of human experience and fascinated by the essential sameness of human beings all over the world.

May I conclude by thanking, in the name of the members of the International Study Group, those who have completed the immense task of compiling these three volumes out of the many and various records of our discussions: Dr Kenneth Soddy, Dr Robert H. Ahrenfeldt, and Miss Mary C. Kidson.

Utrecht   H. C. RÜMKE
January 1964

Editors' Introduction

The Report of the International Study Group on Mental Health, 1961, convened by the World Federation for Mental Health, is being published in three volumes.

Volume I – *Mental Health in a Changing World* – describes the background and work methods of the International Study Group, and presents a summary of the Group's recommendations and an account of the major developments and changes in the world-wide mental health field since the publication in 1948 of *Mental Health and World Citizenship*.

Volume II – *Mental Health and Contemporary Thought* – is concerned with the Study Group's discussions on mental health in relation to the contemporary international scene, on the conceptual background to modern mental health work, and on the implications of modern conditions for professional training and public education in this field.

Volume III – *Mental Health in the Service of the Community* – records the Study Group's discussion of current diagnostic, therapeutic, and prophylactic action in the mental health field, and of the more salient aspects of research.

Originally conceived as one volume, the Report was divided into three volumes for the convenience of those readers who are concerned with a limited sector rather than the whole field of mental health. Like other aspects of social concern, the field of mental health action has widened very considerably in the last few decades. The editors believe that those whose main interest is in the promotion of mental health work may find Volume I the most absorbing of the three; those who are concerned with social problems and the light that the modern sciences of Man can throw on them may find Volume II more to their liking;

and those who are engaged in direct therapeutic work, whether individual or community, may prefer Volume III. For the convenience of readers who do not wish to consult the complete set, the bibliography has been included in each of the volumes.

At the present time it is sometimes said that the method of conference discussion is out of fashion and that it can add little or nothing that is new to its subject. Those who set up the International Study Group on Mental Health, 1961, do not share this view; they consider that the conference discussion has fallen out of favour only among those people who have not understood either its full potentialities or the technical requirements for success. It is readily conceded that a conference may be useless, even harmful, if it is not properly prepared for, and if there is no clear idea of the aims; and, indeed, there is far more to a conference than the mere gathering together of people to talk about a subject. In this volume we have discussed some of the difficulties of people currently engaged in mental health work, and have emphasized the necessity for applying insights gained from modern psychology and allied sciences to the work problems involved. This is true of conferences no less than of other aspects of the work. It would not be reasonable, today, to convene a conference on a mental health subject without bringing to it all the insights available from studies of group dynamics.

It is well recognized that intercommunication is achieved most easily in a group that is homogeneous in terms of age, nationality or culture, educational level, and so on; and with the greatest difficulty when the group is markedly heterogeneous. The International Study Group, 1961, was, by design, interprofessional, transnational, and included a wide age-range. Without a considerable degree of heterogeneity, a study group on transnational mental health questions would be pointless. The inherent difficulties of heterogeneity were, we believe, successfully offset by the specific experience of the Study Group members. The nucleus around which the Study Group was formed was the Scientific Committee of the Federation, the members of which had been in the habit of meeting regularly over a period of about six years for the purpose of studying and writing reports on emerging mental health topics. This group was highly practised in intercommunication; and those members of the International Study Group who were not on the Scientific Committee, though not so closely organized at the outset, also brought with them a wealth of experience of communication across cultural and professional frontiers, and in every case were well known professionally to one or more members of the Scientific Committee.

Thus the Study Group, though apparently heterogeneous, and though coming from many different professions and nations, had in fact achieved a degree of homogeneity of interest in the mental health field before it started its work. The effect of this was quickly visible in the highly integrated work that the Study Group was able to accomplish within a period of two weeks.

Editors of reports are faced with the difficult choice of how far to reproduce verbatim records of discussions and how far to attempt to make a distillate. In the present instance we have tried to achieve a compromise between the extremes. Tape recordings were made of the entire discussions and, in addition, the members themselves had provided a number of working papers and annotations for the editors to draw upon. The main task of the editors has been to arrange the discussions in what appeared to them to be the most logical order, and then to write a considered commentary on the material, illustrating it where appropriate with extracts from the tape recordings and working papers.

The members of the Study Group have voluntarily accepted a group responsibility for what is written in these three volumes. Every member of the Group has had an opportunity to read and comment on the draft and, as far as possible, all the comments received have been acted upon by the editors. That these three volumes represent the agreed Report of the twenty-four members of the Study Group is true in spirit rather than in detail. It is not conceivable that every member agrees with every word that has been written, and in some instances the areas of individual disagreement may be quite wide. Wherever a known area of disagreement or open controversy has been touched upon in the text the editors have attempted to make this clear to the reader.

The editors have been at pains to ensure that the extensive bibliography is accurate and complete up to the summer of 1962. A few books published since that time have been brought to our notice and we have included these under the heading 'Supplementary Titles' but we lacked the facilities to ensure that the list of recent additions is complete.

The editors wish to record their very deep indebtedness to all the members of the Study Group, who have responded so willingly and generously to all requests made for working papers and for criticism and comments on the draft of this Report. A great deal of work has been put into these volumes by a large number of people. We are, of course, most particularly indebted to our Chairman, Professor Dr H. C. Rümke, for his guiding hand throughout the operation and for his highly valued contributions to the compilation of the Report.

We should like to add our own personal note of gratitude to our Editorial Assistant, Miss Mary Kidson, for her immense help throughout, and especially in organizing the very complex material in the later stages of report writing. To her name we would add the names of Miss Elizabeth Barnes, for providing a framework for the first draft of the Report, and Mr Peter Robinson, for his invaluable assistance with the bibliography.

We have found the compilation of this Report a most stimulating and extending experience, and we hope that it will give the reader some notion of the rich field of work to be found in mental health all over the world today.

London   KENNETH SODDY
January 1964   ROBERT H. AHRENFELDT

Note to Volume II

The first of the three volumes that comprise the Report of the World Federation for Mental Health International Study Group of 1961 was mainly devoted to a description of the major trends in the field of mental health since 1948. As remarked in that volume, *Mental Health in a Changing World*, the International Preparatory Commission that preceded the Third International Congress of Mental Health, London, 1948, had made the concept of world citizenship its primary concern. This concern, it can now be seen, had sprung from an emotionally conditioned drive to do something immediately to counteract the evil of the war years.

As an objective, world citizenship is too ill-defined, too complex and diffuse to serve as a focus for work and study in the field of mental health. In its stead the leaders of thought and action in this field have increasingly turned their attention to a more modest but very serious attempt to apply the knowledge and skill gained in professional work on mental health problems to the problems of living in a world suddenly made small by the enormous improvement in communications and more and more crowded by the steep rise in world population.

In this second volume the editors have addressed themselves to the task of writing an interpretative and descriptive free account of the discussions of the International Study Group of 1961 about the application of mental health concepts to the modern world scene, the evolution of the concept of mental health itself, and the style of professional training and public education best suited to present times.

Introductory

The International Study Group of 1961 approached the main item on its agenda by entering into a free-ranging discussion of the general topic of mental health and the contemporary international scene. A social psychologist member of the Group, in opening the discussion, suggested that there are four major problem areas of concern to mental health.

The first is that of international relations proper, as conducted by diplomats and by all those people, official and unofficial, who are in contact with nationals of other countries and who may, by their behaviour, be both contributing to and detracting from mutual understanding and knowledge. There have been a number of recent attempts to improve the quality of understanding between official representatives of countries, notably the conferences on Human Relations in International Secretariats convened by the Carnegie Endowment for International Peace, in cooperation with WFMH; and a series of meetings within the general topic 'The Role of Diplomacy in a Changing World', run on behalf of the American Society of Friends at Clarens, Switzerland, and in Washington. The conviction is growing that something in addition to the conference table may be needed in order to ensure that negotiation can be relied upon to promote international understanding. Many conferences that open promisingly, and with goodwill, end in mutual frustration and in the hardening of the erroneous and hostile stereotypes held by each party about the other. A great deal is now known about the processes of human relations in small groups and there appears to be a vital need for this knowledge to become available and to be applied to diplomatic conferences.

The second major problem area is that loosely referred to as race interaction, though the definition of race in this context is not precise. We are referring to the interaction between different cultural, subcultural, or political groups, both between neighbouring countries and within a single community, and including the very difficult question of ethnic minorities. Recent happenings have underlined the fact that the problem of an ethnic minority in any community is not simply an internal matter, but has profound cross-national implications. Thus the fight to integrate Negro and White children in the schools of the southern states of the USA is watched with deep concern all over the world. The current attempt of the government of the South African Republic to work out its problems of race and colour according to its own specific system of values is causing nothing short of a ferment throughout the rest of Africa and much of Asia, and is also affecting the whole world.

The third problem area is that of social change, which accompanies industrialization and the advance of technology in almost every country. In addition to problems caused by movement of families and change of social groupings, there are the mental health implications of technical assistance, of the peaceful uses of nuclear energy, and of increasing automation.

The fourth problem area is the enormous increase in world population, often referred to as the 'population explosion', though the Study Group had some objection to the use of this term on the grounds of its evocative and pejorative qualities.

All these areas are inherently stressful, a large measure of the foci of stress being found in all levels of human relationships – between people from different countries, cultures, and ethnic groups, and within and between subcultural groups, families, and individuals.

One of the difficulties in the way of understanding these problems is that not enough is known about why different people are capable of interpreting the same phenomena in quite different ways. A social psychologist referred to the current psychological concept of the mirror-image to describe the way in which two people on opposing sides of a question look at each other. Though the analogy applied strictly is misleading, the concept is valuable. Pascal once remarked '*Vérité en deçà des Pyrénées, erreur au delà*' – 'Truth on this side of the Pyrenees, error on the other'. An instructive example of such differences in viewpoint is the contrasting way in which a rapid increase in population may be seen as a blessing by the country concerned and as a curse by a neighbour. In international technical assistance programmes it has been repeatedly seen that aid to a country can be interpreted as a humanitarian gesture by one group and as a gesture of aggression (or 'imperialism' or subversion or whatever is the favoured term of abuse) by another. The different shapes in which reality can appear to individuals on different sides of a question is certainly one of the greatest barriers to understanding.

PART ONE

Mental Health and the Contemporary International Scene

I
Industrialization

One of the most widespread sources of stress in the world today
is industrialization and social development in previously underdeveloped countries. Nearly all countries have problems arising
out of industrialization, ranging from those of a population that
is moving in a single decade from a rural subsistence economy to
an industrial and urban type of life, to those of old-established
industrial societies that are kept in a continuing state of change
by technological advances, automation, and the like.

In a working paper distributed to the Study Group,[1]
Biesheuvel concisely described current developments in much of
Southern Africa. There the progress of industrialization includes
the abandonment of subsistence farming or a peasant way of life
in favour not only of mining, factory, or office work, but also of
work on plantations or estates that produce commercial crops
(timber, fruit, and cotton) in a highly organized manner with the
use of mechanical aids. Thus industrialization does not always
involve a change from rural life to a large and old-established
town; it frequently requires the men to live in compounds away
from their families, or in newly developing townships. It does
not generally permit the maintenance of a village style of community, though theoretically this is possible. In practice, industrialization almost always involves marked changes in habits,
motivation, aspiration, and routines of life.

In Southern Africa, Africans are employed predominantly on
plantations; in mining, building, and construction; and in operative and service work; they supply the bulk of the labour force
below supervisory level. Few Africans are to be found in skilled
trades, and in some places this is due to statutory restrictions.

[1] See *Mental Health in a Changing World*, p. 15.

Africans are now increasingly engaged in clerical, administrative, professional, and commercial work, and also as *entrepreneurs* in transportation, cooperatives, burial societies, catering, and entertainment.

The above picture can be applied *mutatis mutandis* almost anywhere in the world today, wherever industrialization is taking place in previously rural communities. There is always a shortage of skilled tradesmen, and those clerical, administrative, commercial, and middlemen grades that constitute a large bulk of the middle classes in an industrial society lag behind in their development.

PREVENTION OF SOCIAL DESTRUCTION

The Study Group suggested that while it is true that industrialization nearly always destroys the traditional structure of the community into which it is introduced, it has been uncritically assumed that this is inevitable. Hitherto, the precise location of new industrial ventures has generally been determined by factors that do not include any consideration of human relationships. The juxtaposition of raw materials, fuel source, and road, rail, or river communications has usually decided the choice of site. Built on a large scale because of overhead costs, a new factory area becomes a sump into which all detachable manpower and womanpower flow from a wide radius. Acute problems of accommodation and food distribution have to be solved on the spot with no previous planning, and in the resulting chaos all but vestiges of previous social and family structure is apt to be lost.

Is there any valid reason why modern industrial developments should not, in principle, be grafted onto an existing population without dramatically disturbing the existing village social settlement patterns? Modern communications have opened up possibilities which have almost nowhere been sufficiently considered. Roads, railways, harbours, docks, and air strips can be built in a few months; electricity can be carried for hundreds of miles; bus services can vastly increase the radius of daily access to the factory. Automation and mechanical aids increase output in relation to manpower, and so reduce the number of workers required to operate an economically sound unit. No doubt when young men and women travel twenty miles by bus to the local factory social changes will follow. They may prefer to live nearer the factory or they may marry someone from another region who is working in the factory, and in any case they will not maintain an unaltered disciplinary relationship with the village leaders. But such changes would take place over a period of years rather than weeks; they could be foreseen and provided for in town-planning schemes that would at no stage allow a whole community to become rootless, and compelled to improvise new patterns of relationship in a shanty town.

In modern warfare, countries perform remarkable feats in developing new communications. Under the threat of nuclear weapons, countries are planning industrial dispersal into smaller, less economic units, located far from important military targets. What can be done in war and under a potential threat of material destruction could surely be done in order to arrest the social destruction that has already occurred in industrialized countries, and to prevent such destruction from harming newly industrializing countries.

THE NEED TO RAISE PEOPLE'S EXPECTATIONS

The very rapidity of industrial change occurring in previously underdeveloped areas is often blamed for the seriousness of the troubles. The Study Group discussed whether it is not so much the speed of the change that causes difficulties as the nature of the expectations that ordinary people have for themselves. Where a peasant culture has been undisturbed and out of communication with other cultures for a thousand years, no individual can visualize the possibility of change. But such isolation is no longer conceivable anywhere in the modern world, where virtually everyone is aware that processes of change are occurring to other people in other parts of the world. Experience has repeatedly shown that people can pass in a single generation from a peasant culture to a modern industrial community, provided that their expectations

5

for themselves have included the possibility that change may take place in their own case as well as in that of other people, and provided that they do not get bogged down in what an anthropologist described as 'bad habits of social living', represented by slum areas or shanty towns on the edges of large industrial cities.

Social scientists should note that there is now available for study a great deal of evidence concerning the problems in newly independent countries that are embarking on processes of industrial development. It needs also to be realized that while there has been much study of underdeveloped countries by professional observers from other parts of the world, these countries have also been observers, and not entirely passive, of what has been going on elsewhere. In their spontaneous developments can often be seen reflections, not always complimentary, of what they have seen in the people who at that time were acting in a tutelary capacity.

In another working paper, Pacheco e Silva drew attention to the serious vicious circle that exists in so-called underdeveloped countries (the preferred term is now 'developing') in which, in spite of the progress achieved by science and technology, the mass of the population is still struggling for a precarious existence that is quite incompatible with human dignity. In much of Latin America, he considers, the first steps towards promoting the mental health of the inhabitants are inseparable from efforts to raise the general standard of living; the morbidity that goes with undernourishment and substandard living includes physical as well as mental difficulties. Undernourished populations, he points out, are often infested with vermin, malaria, Chagas diseases, trachoma, and other endemic diseases, and many have serious avitaminosis, anaemia, or pulmonary tuberculosis. Under such conditions, maternal and infant mortality and morbidity rates are very high, and expectation of life is short. Not only is disease more prevalent, but resistance to disease is low, the capacity of the population for industrial production is impaired, and the proportion of invalids who are unable to contribute to their own support is unduly high. This combination of adverse circumstances raises very serious mental and physical health problems.

One of the most intractable mental health problems of under-developed areas is how to raise the level of expectation and aspiration of the population so that individuals will expect and, perhaps, demand a higher level of health. A population with many generations' experience of hardship, undernutrition, high morbidity, and short span of life may no more be able to conceptualize change in this direction than the completely isolated peasant population, discussed above, can embrace more general change. Thus, bringing help, in the mental health sense, to such areas raises complex problems, and we know relatively little about the chains of reaction involved. There is a great shortage of personnel with the necessary training to work in these fields, and especially of personnel who understand the problems of specific areas. Least of all do we know how to effect change of attitudes of whole populations where such experiences are traditional.

SOME SOCIAL EFFECTS OF INDUSTRIALIZATION

It appeared to the Study Group that much of the world today resembles a vast but uncoordinated social experiment in the development of industrialization and urbanization among populations that are themselves in a state of constant migration and intermixture. This is particularly true of Latin America whose population, according to recent statistics, has reached some two hundred millions, and is also the fastest-growing population in the world. If the present rate of increase of population is maintained, it will double in less than thirty years.

In his working paper, Pacheco e Silva wrote:

'Notwithstanding the great progress made in many areas of this continent, mainly near the coast, owing to industrialization, mechanization of agriculture, and advances in technology, there are still areas in which the population lives a very primitive life. The great industrial development that has taken place in some parts of Latin America, and particularly the introduction of automation into several heavy industries, has created new problems in the field of mental health. The fast transition from an agrarian to an industrial economy which immediately follows automation has resulted in a great imbalance in social and family life. The simple, bucolic rural life has been replaced by the tension of industrial cities, with their great problems of housing, transportation, and food supply.

The impact of this fast transition has been particularly disturbing to the mental health of the people and has caused disorders of behaviour, drug addiction, neurosis, and psychosis. For this reason, and because of the special circumstances, the introduction of automation into Latin America deserves much more care than the attention that has been given to this problem in other countries. It would be desirable to have intermediate stages to break up the present passage from primitive work conditions directly to an advanced stage of automation.

In the case of Latin America, the population deserves special consideration in some particular aspects in any attempt to plan for the improvement of the mental health of its inhabitants. Unquestionably, the environment influences the personality of man. In order to survive, man is forced to adapt himself to physical, geographical, and social and psychological surroundings.

We can see this dramatically in Latin America; for example, the barometric, climatic, and socio-economic conditions of the Andes plateau have created a human type, with peculiar features of its own, a real climato-physiological variety of the human race. The use of coca in itself is explainable by the extreme conditions of anoxia, which make a "hunger-inhibitor" necessary and a stimulant to prevent fatigue and to make work possible. Similarly, in the north-east of Brazil, the periodical droughts, with their accompanying undernutrition and dehydration, have created also a specific morphological variant. Thus the mental health of people who live in underdeveloped areas is subjected not only to the same noxious influences that act on other populations, but also to other more specific factors.

8

Latin America, in general, is at present one of the great racial laboratories of the world. Ever since its discovery by Europeans, innumerable and successive waves of immigrants of all races and of the most varied nationalities have come to Latin America. With the Amerindians who inhabited the continent at the time of its discovery there have mingled Spanish, Portuguese, French, and Dutch, who, during the struggle for new dominions, came in successive expeditions and stayed for shorter or longer periods. Some of them remained permanently. Later on, the need for labourers to work the soil of this immense territory resulted in African Negroes being brought in.

At the end of the nineteenth century, after the liberation of the slaves, a stream of immigrants arrived from Europe, especially from Italy and the Iberian peninsula. This has not yet ceased, although it has been reduced greatly in recent years. At the beginning of this century the Japanese immigration began, which at certain times reached great proportions. At the same time there was an increasing flow of Syrians, Armenians, Lebanese, Russians, Poles, Germans, Hungarians, Czechs, Lithuanians, Rumanians, Jews, and Chinese, who, attracted by favourable conditions, mainly in Brazil, arrived in considerable numbers.

Thus it happened that the four human races, the red, the white, the black, and the yellow, made an amalgam among themselves, as though in a melting pot. Not only has this produced the most varied physical types, in which sometimes the characteristics of one race, sometimes those of another, have predominated, but it has contributed to the wide diversity of religious creeds, habits, prejudices, customs, and tendencies which have emerged in the descendants of races and peoples of such different origins. This diversity has had a marked influence on the spiritual, cultural, religious, and psychological formation of the various national characters.

The assimilation of immigrants into Latin America presents no major difficulties because of the absence of racial, religious, and class prejudices, or of prejudice of any other kind. This is proved by the number of important positions in politics, liberal professions, commerce, industry, and the armed forces that are already occupied by persons descended from a great variety of races.

It would be a truism to state that extreme poverty and misery have great repercussions on the human mind. Somatic illnesses, physical sufferings, privations, lack of education, and a low standard of living exert undeniable influences in the mental sphere, provoking a great diversity of psychological and psychopathological reactions. And all these factors operate not only on the individual, but at the same time on the family and on the social group.'

In discussing his paper, Pacheco e Silva emphasized the bad individual and social consequences of the tremendous change that is taking place, from subsistence and craft styles of life to a money economy and to automation, without an intermediary period of developing industrialization. The appeal of the new cities as compared with the old way of life has resulted in an overwhelming flood of migration to the towns, and, since accommodation is unobtainable, shanty towns and settlements, with impossible conditions of hygiene and sanitation, have sprung up on the outskirts of industrial cities all over South America. These are conditions that give rise to the 'bad habits of social living' referred to above. But Pacheco e Silva also points out that there is a growing awareness that the conditions existing in these improvised townships are not at all in harmony with modern social developments the world over, with the result that big efforts are now being made to deal with such problems as illiteracy and slum conditions of living.

Processes of change no less massive have been described in other parts of the world where, although the problems of immigration have not been so considerable, the transition from a tribal organization of society to a developing industrial community has involved whole populations. In his working paper, Biesheuvel described some of the phenomena in South Africa during the change from a subsistence to a money economy. He observed that tribal communities living at a subsistence level in pastoral and agricultural communities do not rely even to a slight extent on trade or barter. Today the great majority of tribal communities are being drawn more and more into a money economy. Those who still engage in subsistence farming are becoming dependent in part on money income for cash crops, and on wage-earning for the payment of taxes and the purchase of food supplements, clothing, and household commodities.

Wage-earning involves migration for varying periods of time to large estates, plantations, mines, factories, or to some service occupation. In between these periods subsistence activities may be resumed, but there is a tendency for such families to leave tribal land and settle as labour tenants on large farms, or to become entirely dependent on wages earned in towns. There is an increasing number of landless people in tribal areas.

The absence of a large proportion of adult males for considerable periods causes profound changes in community life:

'Some of the roles performed by them have to be taken over by women. Other functions, especially those related to tribal discussions, counselling, trials, are weakened or fall into disuse. Reduction in the powers of tribal authorities also contribute to this. Ritual observances are reduced in importance or in frequency, again because the whole community is not available to participate in them. Traditional educational practices tend to fall into disuse because the functions for which they were a preparation can no longer be exercised (e.g. the training of Zulu youths in military regiments). On the whole, though, *rites de passage* continue to be observed. The need to make better use of land also alters village life. It necessitates fencing, limitation of cattle, changes in the allocation and management of land, all of which disturb traditional practices and the habits, outlook, beliefs, satisfactions that went with them.'

Biesheuvel also drew attention to the fact that urbanization is relatively new for Africans in Southern Africa, who have had no large indigenous cities to compare with Lagos, Kano, and Timbuctoo. Even the most extensive villages, housing some thousands of people, tend to be impermanent and to remain closely tied to farming pursuits. Processes of urbanization in the Republic of South Africa have resulted in shanty towns and slums which, in recent years, have been tackled by a vigorous policy of rehousing. This, however, has brought in its train certain other problems arising from the policies of racial segregation that are being pursued.

The new townships usually consist of monotonous rows of small, detached houses and, although material conditions are on the whole comparatively good, community life is difficult to foster because the townships are mainly dormitories, with the work being done in the city or surrounding industrial areas. The way of life there has very little in common with traditional village life, and the general lack of education and cultural development in such communities creates serious problems of leadership and hampers the formation of a new cultural tradition.

The state of confusion existing in the minds of the people in these urbanized areas in respect of religion and value systems reflects the wider chaotic picture of change. Biesheuvel stated:

'African religions are animistic and centred on ancestor worship. African thinking is dominated by belief in the pervasiveness of spirit, which links the Deity (a shadowy concept in African cosmologies) through original ancestors, the departed, Man, other living things to the material world in one spiritual continuum. Cause and effect relationships are thought of in terms of interactions between these forces. Different states of being and their power depend on the fluctuating strength of spirit within them. In terms of such a world view, security depends on placation, on spiritual defences and countermeasures. Hence the need to consider the rights of ancestors, in the terrestrial world of here and now, and the significance attaching to magic of all kinds.'

Animistic religions that are centred on ancestor worship are inevitably much influenced by location. Spirits and demons commonly have territories and the spirit of the dead ancestor is usually identified with his grave. As people move away from tribal locations to new towns there is a real danger that they will take with them the anxiety-provoking and more magical aspects of their beliefs, but will be cut off from the capacity to perform the necessary ceremonies to keep the magic good. Hence the magical cults and new religions that spring up in such circumstances, and the great prevalence of superstitions generated by primitive anxiety. It may be noted that movement to new towns is not the only cause of the rise of magical cults.

Among the consequences of social change are new mouldings of personality. Migrant workers have to adjust to two cultures and codes, living now in the one and now in the other. Perhaps even more stressful is having to live and work in two cultures simultaneously, as is the case of the urbanized African who has to adjust to modern industrial standards of work requirements and to a European type of social code at the same time as to the life of the African township. Worst of all, perhaps, is the situation of those whose home life is in a virtually cultureless void where the old institutions have gone and the new ones have not yet evolved. In some slums and shanty towns in Southern Africa, social relationships between Africans, including the marriage relationship, have been described as 'a free for all'.

SOME EFFECTS ON THE FAMILY

The broad social phenomena that we have discussed naturally have their repercussions on the more intimate community and family life of the districts affected. In some ways the family problems of industrialization can be even more acute in societies, as in Southern Africa, where the previous way of life has been settled for some generations, than in the countries of South America, where there is a more general tradition of immigration and of the opening up of undeveloped regions.

There are many examples of countries where processes of industrialization and urbanization have been introduced through the initiative and agency of outsiders into a society that had been previously organized on a peasant – or on a tribal – basis. In the case of a peasant culture there is a traditional extended family pattern with its complex ties of kinship and strong attachments to location; and in the case of a tribal society there are no less complex interpersonal relationships within the tribe on which the security of the whole community is completely dependent. As we have seen, the establishment of factories inevitably creates a drift from agricultural or pastoral life into newly created towns. Usually the sheer fact of population movement makes it impossible for an extended family to keep together or for a tribal organization to persist unimpaired. Thus unless, in the one case, small family units are capable of independent existence, or, in the other case, a whole tribe is involved and can maintain its social structure including its internal relationships, some degree of family and social breakdown is inevitable.

There are many additional reasons why it is highly unlikely that the interpersonal relationships within an uprooted peasant or tribal society can remain unimpaired. Leadership in a newly industrializing community depends on quite other qualities and skills than those characteristic of more traditional social patterns. As the younger members of the uprooted group get to know more about the way of life of other people, and to the extent that they prove more quickly adaptable than the traditional leaders of the community, who are far more identified with the past and much more set in their ways, so the authority structure is bound to disintegrate. On South Africa, Biesheuvel commented:

'In traditional societies, economic insecurities existed only at the communal level, in the form of droughts, crop failures, animal diseases. If anyone suffered from these calamities all suffered alike. There were also protective measures, such as rituals to ensure the growth of crops, and rain-making ceremonies centred on individuals believed to possess special powers. Individual misfortune was always provided for in terms of kinship obligations and the reciprocities between groups. In the cities, however, economic security depends on the getting and holding of a job. It is an individual affair, in which one's own ability and the capriciousness of the employer (in the eyes of the worker) are the determining factors. There is no group ritual, though undoubtedly one can resort to magic as an individual, to increase one's strength, outwit one's enemies, and influence one's employer.

Some of the traditional reciprocity remains in the cities, but it works against, rather than in favour of, the establishment of a sense of economic security, at least for the wage-earner. An ever-widening circle of relatives tends to gather around the worker who prospers, but few of them are able to do anything in return for him, should he lose his job. A Congo politician recently declared that a group of Congolese workers had declined an increase in wages for fear that knowledge of this would bring another wave of relatives from the country to share their good fortune.

In most traditional societies people felt reasonably safe from the risk of accidental injury or assault. Industrial and urban life is far more hazardous. The violence that prevails in townships is a common theme in African literature and in stories written in response to projection tests. Migrant workers from tribal areas are known to prefer employment in the mines to industrial work, because mine compounds provide sheltered living conditions and save them from the dangers associated with township life. This is also a factor which deters them from bringing their families to the towns. Living dangerously may well have its attractions for those venturesome spirits who seek excitement and achievement in otherwise drab lives. But for the majority the threat of assault, robbery, and the attention of gangs who exact "protection money" adds considerable insecurity to daily life.

The rural African is more defenceless against disease than the city dweller, but education has not greatly altered his attitude towards illness. Although he knows some of the agencies whereby illness comes about, and learns how to protect himself against these, for the majority the ultimate cause still remains the evil intentions of another person or ancestor, who has manipulated the precipitating pathogenic factors. These fears persist, despite education even to an advanced level.

Family Life

Cultural change has had more far-reaching effects on family life than on any other institution. In villages, migratory labour practices have undermined marital fidelity. Kinship bonds and responsibilities retain, however, much of their vigour, and the child still grows up in an extended family which ensures its normal development along traditional lines. Elsewhere, the family persists in an attenuated form which, in the cities, reduces itself generally to father, mother, and children.

In tribal societies marriage involved a contract between kinship groups, rather than between individuals. A complicated system of reciprocities was made real and enforceable through the transfer of lobola (bride-price) cattle. Lobola is still an essential ingredient of city marriages, even those solemnized according to Christian rites; but it has radically altered its function and no longer has the same binding force, as it is paid in money rather than in cattle, and involves individuals rather than their families. Divorce and desertion, virtually non-existent in tribal societies, are now common. Still more common are temporary unions engaged in by women who keep house for migrant males and who are left to take care of the successive offspring. Illegitimacy is rife at all social levels. Remnants of traditional child-rearing practices linger on; but they are no longer functional for the new urban societies, nor can they be effectively applied outside the extended family where each member plays a particular formative role. The new urban family frequently lacks the stability, attitudes, and understanding to be able to induce conformity to Western codes. As a result, social disorder and delinquency have become serious problems, for which school education and the Christian church have not been able to provide fully effective remedies. Finally, there are the old people to be considered. Their secure position in tribal society no longer obtains in the cities. The weakening of kinship bonds, housing problems, and the fact that what they eat and wear must be bought increases the probability that at some stage they will be left destitute.

Personality Development

The social personalities of Africans in tribal communities were typically tradition-directed. In such personalities, "culture controls behaviour minutely" (667) and shame is a more potent agent of conformity than guilt. Individuality is less a matter of attainment and aspirations, which are largely conditioned by traditional social roles, than of temperament make-up. Such personalities do not develop under the new urban conditions. Nor are conditions favourable for the growth of inner-direction, which depends on the inculcation of a well-defined value system by means of powerful parental influences. Elsewhere it has been shown that as a result of the formlessness of township society, the confusion of its values, and the relative absence or negative nature of pressures towards conformity in the home, personalities emerge which are more nearly *id*-directed, moved greatly neither by shame nor by guilt, and which are restrained, if at all, only by fear of immediate physical retribution (570). The violence that characterizes township life provides some evidence in support of this hypothesis.

Rae Sherwood in a hitherto unpublished study of African clerical and professional workers has shown that in African middle-class society (where presumably the conditions under which children are reared are more favourable) the trend is towards the other-directed personality type, sensitive to the actions, wishes, aspirations, and approval of its contemporaries (in this case the Whites, whose approval is a condition for security and advancement).

Riesman says of the other-directed personality: "As against guilt and shame controls, though of course these survive, one prime psychological lever of the other-directed person is diffuse anxiety." The addition of elements of racial discrimination, which creates a conflict of interests and places barriers between the African middle class and its white peer groups, tends to increase the strength of this anxiety.'

As the illustrations above have suggested, processes of social change that create a volume of migration are almost bound to break up traditional community and family patterns. In a working paper, Soddy noted that the industrial revolution had its origin in precisely those areas in which the families were most inherently capable of survival as small, independent, so-called 'nuclear' units. In England, for example, where the early stages of the industrial revolution developed most rapidly, the social norm of having only one married couple in each household had been widespread since the Middle Ages.[1] In this setting, when the time came for the young married couple to leave the farm and go to the newly developing town to get factory work, no new principle of social relationship was involved. But there is another aspect of change of family life caused by developing industrialization that may precede a more obvious break-up of families when the young married couple migrates to a distant town. This more subtle process of change is set in motion when work begins to be separated from home. In a peasant subsistence economy, practically the whole population works within easy walking distance of their homes. When the father of the family starts working at a place which takes him away from his family during the day, the whole character of family life is immediately changed. If his absences are extended to several days at a time or even months, as is very commonly the pattern, the effects on family life are even greater.

It may be observed that industrialization has caused less evidence of social disorganization in Great Britain than elsewhere, in spite of its early appearance and the high intensity of industrialization achieved. During the latter part of the nineteenth century, industrialization spread as it were by contagion into the cultures in which the families were still living in a peasant type

[1] See Laslett, P., 1965. *The World We Have Lost*. London.

of organization, with a rigid extended structure, and it has been in this type of setting that evidence of social disorganization has been greatest. Soddy wrote:

'It is a reasonable conclusion that the extended family is comparatively vulnerable to conditions that impede or prevent the smooth functioning of the complex family unit or familiar living, and that this will be particularly true in times of rapid social change. This conclusion is of particular importance at the present time when in many countries of Africa, South America, Asia, and some parts of Europe, communities with a traditional agrarian culture are being pitched in a couple of decades into a state of almost complete industrialization.

At the First Asian Seminar on Mental Health and Family Life in the Philippine Islands, December 1958, much anxiety was expressed by participants about the so-called "breakdown of family life" that was foreseen whenever industrialization occurred (which is almost everywhere today). It seemed a widespread assumption there that when collateral branches of the family are no longer available for mutual support, this is a disaster which might well overwhelm and distintegrate the family structure and, through that, society as a whole. The delegates did not credit that there were enough resources in the human relationships of the small biological family group to provide security. A symptom of this anxiety was the widespread propaganda in favour of the extended family in the Philippines at the time. A typical slogan, specially printed for sticking to car windscreens, and much displayed, was "the family that prays together, stays together". The apparent assumption here is that family cohesiveness and solidarity are essential prerequisites of social survival in an age felt to be insecure, dangerous, and menacing.'

Soddy pointed out that the fact that the extended family is vulnerable to the type of change that causes a break-up of its communal life does not imply that the nuclear family has no vulnerable aspects of its own. For example, when the mother of a young family that is living independently suffers a breakdown in health, who is to take her place? Even if grandparents and collaterals are living within reach they may well be comparative strangers to the young children. In times of stress, the nuclear family society is also inclined to value family cohesion very highly, and as evidence of this can be cited the use of the current slogan 'togetherness'. Such feelings of need for support from relatives often create a nostalgic attitude towards the supposedly more settled relationships of older times, which may have little to do with objective history.

Biesheuvel observed that the conditions in which the traditional extended family is most vulnerable are characteristic to a striking degree of transitional urban communities in Southern Africa. In these conditions it is very difficult to plan effective preventive and therapeutic measures for children in need. There are, for example, grave practical problems in the way of making use of child guidance services in the unstable social context of the broken-down extended family, in which the traditional chains of responsibility with the family have disintegrated. He asked the following questions:

'(i) Who acts as the referral agency for the wayward and disturbed child when the family itself has more or less disintegrated, or when the child does not go to school, or when the school is overcrowded or the teacher untrained and too hardpressed to notice that anything is wrong?

(ii) To whom must remedial counselling be given if the father is not available, and the mother is at work or overburdened or unable to grasp the nature of what is now being asked of the family?

(iii) Who sees that the treatment plan is followed?

(iv) How can even simple prophylactic measures be applied effectively when even the rudiments of sound education as understood in the new context of life are not being given in the community?'

He commented that this situation is endemic in many parts of

Africa today, and is not just a matter of isolated cases. It calls less for individual than for social therapeutic measures. Perhaps this complex problem can be tackled only at a government-planning level by people with a sophisticated grasp of the reality of the psychosocial forces involved in such stark social changes.

2

Social Change

THE NATURE OF CHANGE

Although many of the phenomena of change have been exhaustively described, this should not be allowed to obscure the fact that we have comparatively little idea of the basic nature of change. It may be said that so little is known about the effects of change that the present generation is not able to prepare children to meet anticipated change in the future, and realization of this inability may well be a source of anxiety and tension in family life today.

The Study Group set out to examine this matter a little further, and started by attempting to draw a distinction between changes in man's relationship with himself and changes in the relationship between man and his works. The observation is commonly made that although man's inventive genius has resulted in vast changes in his works, there has been little change in his relationship with himself. Human nature is popularly deemed to be more or less unchanging, but that this may not be strictly true can be illustrated by a traditional story in French school textbooks: Marshal Turenne found that he was trembling during a battle, and said to himself, 'Carcass, you dare tremble!' At first sight this might appear to be a form of introspection, even of possession of insight, but a psychiatrist at the Study Group suggested that an alternative interpretation might be legitimate – that it represents a detachment, an increasing of the distance between the volition and the body. Such control of physical reactions by the will has been traditionally taught through the ages, especially to children. It contrasts strongly with later attitudes towards anxiety and the concept of 'war neurosis'. More commonly, the modern attitude is to seek to decrease the distance between the volition and more primitive emotional reactions. A value is now set on self-identification as a whole personality and the full acceptance of that part of oneself – to be compensated for if necessary – which Marshal Turenne would have regarded as a weakness to be extirpated.

Inasmuch as such insights and attitudes are now comparatively widespread in the population, and not merely limited to a few students of human psychology, this is evidence of a change in the nature of man and a shrinking of the distance between man and himself. In contrast, the distance between man and what he creates appears to be increasing. A traditional craftsman used to become more or less completely identified with his occupation with his whole personality and, at least in the case of a craftsman in a subsistence economy, there may have been very little to the individual's life apart from his work. In a modern industrial society man has been getting progressively more detached from his work. Relatively few people today, mostly limited to the small professional classes, become completely identified with their work. The more general attitude is to regard work as something apart from the real life and interests of the individual, something that provides only the means whereby the individual may express his personality for himself – hence the importance of so-called leisure time and hobbies.

There are very many other examples of changes now taking place in the life of modern society which relate to improvements in communication and to differences in work relationships. As a member of the Study Group remarked: this is not merely a matter of radio, television, aircraft, or automation; these innovations do not themselves create the problem, but they materially alter the interrelationships between people. Temporal and spatial structures are modified by man's endeavours, but it is the profound change in internal and external reference systems that these may cause that can constitute the problem, through the very considerable effect that it can have on the orientation and sense of identity of the individual. The Mexican peasant who, only a decade ago, may have had to spend six days on muleback in order to reach the capital can do the same journey in one hour today, if he can afford the fare. In some respects we are now living almost at the level of fairy stories, of seven-league boots and magic carpets, of giants and magicians. It is progressively more difficult for the ordinary man to preserve a sense of proportion and of a continuous interrelationship with his environment.

Much that is thought and written about change, including, perhaps, the preceding paragraphs, leaves an impression on the reader that stasis is regarded as the norm and change as something to which the individual has to make an adaptation, at the cost of some stress. In fact this view of the nature of change can be justified, and then only to a limited extent, only if a long-term view extending over the human life-span is taken of the community as a whole. It is true that there have been communities at certain periods in history in which the rate of discernible change has been very slow indeed. But this view of change can never be applied to the individual, who, by the very facts of growth and development, the evolution of family relations and work, the processes of ageing and death, is in a state of continuous change. There is no static norm.

We would prefer to approach this question from the theoretical standpoint that change not only is an inescapable necessity for every human being; it is also a major source of benefit and satisfaction. In every culture the tiny infant derives his major satisfactions from incorporating into his own being the environmental experiences that his mother mediates to him. The most important of these is food, but there is a host of innovations and learning experiences that the mother passes on to the child.

In the case of young children the effects of this programme of innovation and change are obvious and vast. Not only do the great majority enjoy change, look forward to it and seek it, but they themselves become different people in the process of absorption of change. We are not aware of the existence of any culture in which it is possible to set a time-limit on the capacity of human beings to get satisfaction from change and development, but there are wide variations in the respective capacities of individuals belonging to different cultures, of different individuals in the same culture, and in the capacity of the same individual at different periods of life, to accept, absorb, enjoy, and develop with change. These variations occur both in the scope and time relations of the changes involved, and in relation to the origins and modes of introduction of the innovations.

There is no body of satisfactory evidence that can give a guide as to which people can absorb what degrees of change and at what speed or with what intermediate gradations of change. We certainly cannot assume that in a particular case an abrupt radical change produces more strains for the individual than a series of graduated partial changes, though public practice often appears to reflect this assumption. The Mexican peasant of our example represents a midway position between the modern city-dweller who is accustomed to fast surface transport and the man from the tribal community who has no technical aids to locomotion, not even a wheel or shoes. Does the first flight by aeroplane represent greater stress on the man coming from a simpler environment, a remote peasant community, or a modern city? No single answer can be given to this question, because of wide differences in the situation of the three individuals concerned. The tribal man has no standards by which to judge the new experience, but he is not cut off from the magical components of his philosophy of life and he might be readier to take the aeroplane ride than the peasant, whose freedom of attitude might have been restricted by centuries of unvarying custom. On the other hand, the peasant would already have heard of the existence of air transport and might have been introduced to it favourably; whereas the city dweller might be more aware of its dangers and difficulties.

We have suggested above that the alterations that occur in human relationships as a result of social change may be of more significance than the actual innovations themselves. The air journey would take the tribal man into a totally unfamiliar world, but unlike the peasant he would have acquired no fixed habits of living in a complex society that might interfere with his adaptation. The peasant would necessarily approach the new environment with his capacity for flexible reaction reduced by past experience. The six-day mule-ride would take the peasant out of his familiar environment and force him to make a continuous effort of personal adaptation, with the objective of the big city always in his mind. Thus the journey would itself be an adaptive process that would leave him in a frame of mind very different from that in which he would disembark from the aircraft after a mere hour's flight. However, it might require only one or two repetitions of the experience to make the short air journey as adequate a preparation as the long mule journey.

RATE OF SOCIAL CHANGE

It is commonly held, in respect of the effects of change on the community, that social change is more likely to be achieved successfully if the rate of change is slow, and that the factor on which success depends most is the speed at which the population can adapt to new things. On the other hand, in the case of previously undisturbed communities suddenly exposed to change during the violent upheavals contingent upon World War I, it was repeatedly demonstrated that it is possible for a society to move from a Bronze-Age social and technological pattern to a modern community in the course of twenty-five years.

In a working paper, Mead emphasized that in the field of social change the technological methods in use are themselves changing rapidly, which calls for the revision of many previously held ideas. In the early 1950s, for example, it was still quite usual to devote a great deal of attention in community projects in undeveloped areas to such requirements as the laborious persuasion of leaders in each village to supply their share of the labour if a road was to be built. Current methods of road-building with powered earth-moving equipment require no such detailed village-by-village participation. Instead, a different set of problems of adjustment have been created, which are concerned not so much with local community responsibility as with the sudden easy accessibility of previously distant urban contacts. Mead wrote:

'In general, ten years ago, most students of human behaviour felt that slow change was, at least in many ways, better than rapid change, as far as the mental health of those who were involved in the change was concerned. This orientation meant that the mental health sciences – psychiatry, anthropology, sociology, social psychology, etc. – were often arrayed against the economists and technologists who were pushing for rapid change. This position was based on experience of change situations in which the changes were not desired by the populations experiencing them, but were thrust upon them by colonial powers, by industrial expansion, by reformers and modernizers who were seen as alien. Accumulating experience since that time suggests that, instead of proposing slow change, we should propose various methods of transformation in which the entire set of living habits of a people is changed to another level, when they move on from one country to another, from country to city, or from a preliterate to a literate way of life. In our earlier work (504) we stressed the mental health problems of the second generation, reared under conditions of extreme change, where their parents had had the benefit of a more stable upbringing than they had had themselves. However, more recent work suggests that this picture is considerably oversimplified, and we must consider that much of the damage is done by uneven change – slow in some respects, fast in others – and the formation of patterns of behaviour and associated character structures, which are themselves compromise formations between the old and the new. Sometimes very rapid, across-the-board change, especially when it is spontaneous and involves all generations (505), may be able to bypass these temporary maladaptive habits, such as those involved in slum-living, where people learn how not to live in a city by being forced to occupy quarters which are themselves inadequate and often not even designed for the purposes for which they are later used (531). We also know much more about special types of change, such as those involved in the adjustment of young Chinese to Westernization (16).'

PLANNING AND SOCIAL CHANGE

There is still far too little known about planning in respect of problems of technical change and rural-urban migration. The government of Ghana showed an encouraging initiative during the building of the Volta river dam, which involved bringing in, for a period of four years of settled work, workers who had previously lived in the bush. The government sought expert advice on the social and mental health of the workers. In recommending an extension of such action, the Study Group felt that a useful role could be served by the formation of national committees of experts in the human sciences to take part in planning, from the inception of every major scheme that might have social repercussions. This is especially pertinent when major social changes are taking place in countries developing from a previously settled existence into a modern industrial community. Under these conditions it is more than overdue that consideration of mental health aspects should be habitual to the thinking of social planners.

Concern for mental health during the phase of planning should not be centred exclusively on those who are making the change, but should also include provision for the mental health problems of those who find it difficult to make the change and who may cling to the old way of life. It is possible that in some communities the most serious mental health problems may be found among those who are representative of the old way of life rather than among the people who are changing.

In some countries with a long history of industrial development, the planning of new towns has not always shown sensitivity to social balances, as, for example, when new housing has been allocated on a basis of giving houses to those who have the greatest need for accommodation, irrespective of social role, so that whole new areas have been created where the social grouping is quite atypical of the surrounding districts. This is almost bound to set up points of potential tension in the society.

Planning should also take into consideration what is likely to happen to the next generation – to the children who are brought up in these new communities, which may be so very different from the communities in which their own parents grew up. For example, it has been the experience in some of the older residential housing estates on the outskirts of London, established during the large slum-clearance projects of the interwar period, that members of the first generation of those born and brought up on the estates have not been allowed to settle there on marriage. The housing authority has preferred to replace families as they move out with other families from current slum-clearance projects. It appears that the housing authority has not considered the likely effect on the community of creating what will amount to a permanent long-term transit camp, with an almost complete fragmentation of family networks as far as that community is concerned.

In the case of newly developing countries, the first-generation problems arising out of lack of mental health planning are likely to occur much earlier and in a more acute form. A striking example was described to the Study Group of a difficulty encountered during the development of oil production in the Sahara desert. Much of the labour employed in the early stages was recruited from nomadic tribes, and more or less permanent settlements were created. In the course of a few years, the increasingly technological nature of the employment as oil production proceeded and the habitual restlessness of a previously nomadic people combined to cause the return to the desert of considerable numbers of employees. It was found that, whereas the adults in most cases readjusted to the nomadic life without difficulty, the problems of their children tended to be intractable.

It is clearly impossible for human beings to maintain life in the desert without having learnt how to do so, and the training of the children in nomadic tribes is prolonged and rigorous. When a previously nomadic desert tribe becomes settled, both the oral transmission and the practical demonstration of the traditional ways of desert life are abruptly and completely interrupted. The children literally do not know how to live in the desert.

Admittedly, the above example is a very special case, but it illustrates the important point that, when individuals of more than one generation are required to adapt to profound social change at the same time, the reactions may be many and various. Even the unfavourable reactions, such as excessive anxiety, excessive conformity to the change, rejection of the change, apathy, withdrawal, or aggressive hostility may be found intermingled among the different generations of members of one family. There is a great need for a more informed approach in respect of mental health matters in projects of social development.

Where, as sometimes happens, the entire cultural matrix of a peasant economy begins to disintegrate under the various processes set in train by the impact of modern technological civilization, the degree of social adjustment that may result among those belonging to the culture may be dependent upon the amount of security that individual members can find in the enlarging opportunities of which they have become aware. It appeared to the Study Group that, for example, wherever in Southern Africa policies of discrimination have had the result that people of one type of origin have been able to see that many opportunities are closed for themselves, but not for certain other·people in the community, the resulting social maladjustment is bound to be severe and persistent. This social maladjustment affects not only those who are suffering from discrimination, but also the discriminators, who are inevitably impelled by their own actions to maintain and even to increase the tensions that are causing the social maladjustment. Thus the situation can arise, and we believe it has arisen, where the policy-makers and the classes that are discriminated against are both caught up in a pressure of activity that relates not to the reality situation and the needs of the community as a whole, but to the relationship that exists between the two sides.

MANAGEMENT OF SOCIAL CHANGE

It is an integral part of planning of social change that action be preceded and accompanied by surveys in order that some objective control be kept on social policies. As a result of surveys it was shown that after a big rehousing project in Lima, Peru, there were fewer visits to doctors and less drug addiction, alcoholism, and crime – information of extreme value in getting a community to finance further programmes of social amelioration.

Such programmes would be greatly facilitated by the development for a given community of indices of mental health, mental illness, and social disorganization. As discussed later in this volume there is little exact knowledge of such possible indices at present, beyond rather crude suggestive indications, such as high suicide and mental-illness rates reported in connexion with big population movements, which, there may be reason for thinking, had been engendered by insecurity, and the prejudice and discrimination encountered by migrant groups. It is possible that indices might be developed from among the statistics of incidence and prevalence of the so-called psychosocial and psychosomatic stress disorders.

The role of subcultural groups in the production of social disorganization needs more elucidation. It is a commonplace in communities well equipped with social agencies to find that 5 or 6 per cent of families produce a disproportionate amount of sociomedical difficulty. The Study Group considered that, on the whole, social disorganization is not directly connected with processes of industrial change as such, and that it is possible that in any given society the lowest 5 per cent on the socio-economic scale could be regarded as a subcultural group in terms of that society. Whether the existence of a subcultural group gives rise to social problems is a question that depends on many other factors, including those of social change.

WORK ATTITUDES AND MOTIVATION

In a working paper, Biesheuvel commented that, in a subsistence economy where, broadly speaking, men and women work only as much as is necessary to maintain life, there is no sharp distinction between work and other communal activities. In an industrialized society with a money economy, work is far more than a physiological necessity of life; it satisfies numerous other needs – social, individualistic, and moral. Biesheuvel continued:

'How have Africans met this transition? A. H. Maslow has put forward a need-hierarchy theory which postulates that higher needs are not activated until those below them are adequately satisfied. The four needs in this hierarchy from low to high are: physiological or safety needs; the need to belong; ego needs (self-esteem and other-esteem); and self-actualization (the need to realize all one's potentialities). One can see the development of this need-hierarchy almost phylogenetically as the African worker proceeds from the migrant, through the urbanized operative, to the skilled, white-collar, or professional stages. Attitude studies carried out by Hudson, Glass, Cortis, and R. Sherwood at the National Institute for Personnel Research show that the migrant mineworker remains a peasant with no work ambition other than to satisfy the basic needs for food, clothing, and cattle for bride-price purposes. The fully urbanized operative, however, is concerned with security at a rather higher level. He places "liability to be dismissed at short notice or to be laid off" top of a list of job dissatisfactions. Though both he and the migrant labourer stress the importance of considerate treatment by supervisors and managers, they mention the desirability of good relations with fellow employees, or of being consulted about conditions of service (participation, other-esteem) far less often than do White daily-paid employees at a higher level in the same factories. In an African clerical group, however, service towards the community and pleasant human relations with both management and fellow-workers are placed first among major causes of job satisfaction. The clerks attach rather less importance to self-actualization motives (intrinsic interest in the job, learning new skills, self-expression). These satisfactions are mentioned most frequently by a professional African group.

The implications of these studies are that, as Africans get more deeply involved in an economy of the Western type, so they acquire step by step the work attitudes appropriate to such an economy. They acquire similar needs, but are exposed to somewhat different frustrations and anxieties whenever racial distinctions place them in a marginal position or impose restrictions on their advancement. Women workers present a special case, because of the subordinate position which they occupy in many African tribes, and the new powers which employment confers on them. Work has provided various means of emancipation which sometimes take a curious form (e.g. payment by the woman herself of bride-price to secure a claim to children, husband's fidelity, or future parental support in case of husband's desertion).'

Considerable new problems of work motivation are being raised by increasing mechanization leading to automation. It has been demonstrated ever since the introduction of power machinery in the early period of the industrial revolution that workers have regarded increasing mechanization with anxiety that is very much deeper than the fear that they may suffer economic privation through loss of employment. Mechanization has always been felt as a threat to the potency and usefulness of the individual or, in Maslow's terms, to his need to belong, to self-esteem and the esteem of others, and to self-realization. Yet, as Veil pointed out in a working paper, there is no justification for adopting either the attitude that machines will deprive man of his rights or the contrary one, that man must necessarily be overburdened by increasing demands of work. Veil wrote:

'We know that the simultaneous discovery of new sources of energy and new mechanical devices is going to make profound changes in the role of workers. Occupational hierarchies and qualifications, interpersonal relations, etc., will not remain the same as they are today. Nor will the motor, psychomotor, and intellectual operations be the same. The nature of the material and emotional relationships that the worker has with his working material, the product, his tools, his fellow-workers, his supervisors, his employer, and his family will change. The

33

hours of work, the amount of leisure and the form this takes, and in a more general way the worker's attitude to the spending of time will also evolve. It is impossible to foresee whether this evolution will represent to some extent a regression towards the slavery of antiquity, or, on the contrary, a liberation from traditional forms of servitude. This will partly depend on the nature of the new relationships that will be formed between employers, wage earners, and public authorities. We can reach no firm conclusions on this point either, but the question must be raised.

It may be worth recalling that, however important the technological factors may be, they always lead back in the last analysis to human factors. Automation (like mechanization and the division of work which preceded it historically) is neither good nor bad in itself. It will become what man makes of it. It is for those of us here to help mankind to develop it for the best.'

LEISURE

In the highly industrialized countries the question of leisure is assuming greater dimensions in people's minds. It may be felt that preoccupation with leisure represents almost a full circle of progress from a subsistence economy into industrialization. In the former, leisure is accepted as what might be described as 'the continuous phase' and work is regarded as a means of returning to leisure. During industrialization it becomes the assumption that work is the aim and duty of mankind, and in the countries that pioneered industrialization it has been the experience everywhere that leisure has had to be fought for, step by step, by legislation, by the invocation of humanitarian sentiments, and, most powerfully, by the workers themselves. This continuous process has led towards the shortening of working hours which, in most instances, has been resisted on the side of the employers, not only because of a supposed loss of production, but also because of infringement of a set of moral assumptions.

It is a measure of the degree to which moral issues have become caught up in this whole field that people are almost everywhere prepared to make moral judgements about the value of leisure and the wise use of leisure. There is a widespread fear in many quarters that if a high proportion of the population has a great deal of unoccupied time on its hands, there will be considerable social, if not moral, danger.

There are a number of divergent trends here. Increasing mechanization and automation are tending to reduce working hours, to which situation more and more workers are reacting by taking a second job in their so-called leisure hours. In the case of some professions where standard remuneration has not kept pace with rising prices, this reaction has been determined primarily by money needs, but it is often the case that people take on a second job because they do not know what to do with the time they previously gave to work. It is often stated that automation is likely to mean that fewer people will get satisfaction from their work, and that this may tend to unbalance the whole structure of human relations in industry. This is largely a speculation on which the evidence is at present unclear. It is possible that automation may tend to increase the distance between the comparatively small group of very highly skilled technocrats, who will build, service, and maintain the machines and who will be virtually irreplaceable, and those who will operate the machines without technological knowledge and who will be easily replaceable. The task of the latter will probably entail long periods of physical inactivity combined with a responsibility for watchfulness – conditions that will create a new type of working stress on the majority. In addition, those workers of below-average intellectual and educational level, whose main work satisfaction has previously been obtained from physical movement and bodily achievement, may not be able to get the satisfactions they need in a fully automated industrial society.

RETIREMENT

The Study Group expressed considerable dissatisfaction with the attitude towards retirement policies in most industrialized countries. There is a strong case for investigating the possibilities of arrangements for staging or grading retirement; and there is a great need for clearer understanding about retirement on the part of both management and workers. One member of the Study Group referred to the occurrence of death soon after retirement as 'the real mortal danger of retirement'. We need to get much more exact information about death rates in relation to sex, occupation, and retirement.

The strictly local significance of such studies is recognized. In cultures, subcultural groups, or social classes in which the family is organized on an extended pattern, the old people may well gain all the support that they need from the family group. But in societies with a nuclear form of family organization there is a strong case for the early preparation of the middle-aged generation for the problems of retirement of the elderly. Where it is the usual practice for young adults to establish their own separate homes upon marriage and to retain only such contact with their parents as may be determined by ties of mutual affection, there may be a strong resistance from both parties to the resumption of any dependent relationship, with the roles reversed, after a lapse of thirty years, especially where long distances have resulted in infrequent contacts during the intervening years. In this style of family life the individual's first twenty years are spent in an atmosphere that encourages growth towards complete independence from parents, which is the goal of parents and children, alike. The return thirty years later to a reversed dependency relationship, of aged parent on middle-aged offspring, requires a radical change of attitudes for which neither party is psychologically prepared. We need to know more about how to anticipate and provide for the needs of old people living in a society with a nuclear style of family life, in an era of increasing expectation of life and therefore of an increasing proportion of old people. It would be far better to make suitable arrangements with the provision and cooperation of the family than to improvise in an emergency as is so often the case at present. The involvement of adolescent children whose parents are facing these problems in relation to the grandparents is an additional important field for mental health study.

INDICATIONS OF MORE MORBID DEGREES OF STRAIN

Signs of stress indicating more morbid degrees of strain in an industrializing population are likely to be at their greatest where rapid development has been imposed by external circumstances upon a community which previously had a low standard of living. It is likely that many of the more florid stress disorders will have been widely prevalent in the population before the changes occurred and may relate to the disastrous effect of climatic vagaries upon a society living by a subsistence economy.

A South American psychiatrist pointed out that, for example, in the north-east of Brazil, where prolonged droughts occur periodically and the population suffers intermittently from dehydration, there is a high incidence of mental illness due to nutritional deficiency and cerebral anaemia, notably states of confusion associated with polyneuritis, as described by Korsakov. Further, the hardship suffered often causes the inhabitants to seek escape in drugs, and there are high rates of cocaine addiction in Peru, of marihuana addiction in Brazil, and of alcoholism throughout Latin America and particularly in Chile.

Drugs appear to have an increased upsetting effect when the constitution is debilitated, especially after a low-protein diet, and their use is associated with a high incidence of acute psychosis of a hebephrenic type, pathological ecstasy, and impulsive aggressive or homicidal acts. Similar psychotic states have been reported common during the wanderings of migrant populations, and more frequently when a migrant population is exposed to a more highly industrialized type of life. Under these conditions there is a relatively high incidence of puerperal psychosis, which is associated with malnutrition, lack of skilled assistance, and high infection rates. Naturally, a high infantile mortality rate will add to the emotional problems of the parents.

Other mental sequelae include a high prevalence of mental deficiency, epilepsy, and endemic encephalitis and meningitis with neurological and psychological sequelae. In these populations therefore there is an unduly high proportion of children who are ineducable in normal schools, which creates a considerable social problem, especially where there are not enough educational facilities for everyone. Measures for the care and rehabilitation of defectives and the chronically psychotic are very difficult to implement under such conditions.

3
Individual Change

The spread of universal compulsory school attendance has brought many problems both to old-established industrial communities and to tribal societies in the first generation of urbanization. In respect of the latter, in a working paper Biesheuvel remarked that the modern school differs from the 'initiation school' of the tribal society in that the emphasis is on individual achievement rather than on preparation for group activities and tribal roles. Thus the child brought up in a tribal society finds himself in a very foreign atmosphere in a modern school. Biesheuvel comments that the African pupil generally addresses himself to school with great determination and, being aware of his handicaps and of the importance of success in examinations, tends to rely predominantly on memory when understanding does not help him. This may place him in a vulnerable position which may get worse higher up the educational scale. This problem was discussed at the CCTA/CSA meeting of specialists on 'The basic psychology of African and Madagascan populations' at Tananarive in 1959 (512).

Problems of a similar order, though manifested in more complex forms, have been created by the spread of compulsory education in established industrial societies. In a number of countries there is nearly a century of experience of universal elementary education, and in these countries the idea of going to school and something of what it entails are very familiar to the children well before they reach school entry age. Three generations ago schools set out mainly to teach the 'three Rs'—reading, writing, and arithmetic—information was kept to a minimum and technical education scarcely touched upon. The majority of

39

children left school while they were pre-adolescent, and in many ways the most important part of their education began after they had left school. All over the world in the last half-century, education in schools has become progressively more academic, concerned with more information, more technical. It has demanded a progressively higher level of ability and effort, a fact that has been recognized in some educational systems in which intelligence and attainment barriers are used to limit the later scholastic education of those who do not pass certain tests at an earlier age.

The Study Group was hardly concerned in this context with such complicated educational questions as segregation by ability of children for education. Our wish here is to draw attention to the fact that the life and experience of the classroom have now been prolonged quite a long way into adolescence for the whole population of modern industrial societies and for much of the rest of the world also.

There are many problems involved: for example, have the traditional school methods based on the 'three Rs' given place to the new kinds of attitude required? A more immediate problem is the effect on the children's development of the invasion of adolescence by school, particularly in respect of the population that lies below the intellectual mean.

We have made several references to the anxiety felt in some countries about the behaviour of teenage youth, and the question of what the educational system should do in the face of rising figures of delinquency. However, delinquency is only one possible sign of the existence of a disturbance among youth. Only a proportion of disturbed youth will act out their anxiety in maladjustment and delinquent behaviour; there may be many others whose anxiety takes a more in-turning form but who are nevertheless disturbed.

It needs to be asked how far society is failing these young people in trouble, and how far one ought to look for other causes, perhaps in the young people themselves. An educational psychologist in the Study Group remarked that, as far as the United

Kingdom is concerned, experience is showing that where a school develops a vocational bias, that is, not a wholly vocational training but a normal school curriculum with opportunity for vocational training, those children who are below the mean in intelligence may be better able to develop a clear and foreseeable vocational goal. This has tended to increase the proportion of children who are willing to stay on after passing the age for compulsory schooling (in 1961 the first possible school-leaving age in the United Kingdom was fifteen). The same is true of those schools that develop a high morale through the involvement of individual children in group activities and the group role rather than in education on an individualistic basis.

The question of whether the schools have been successful in extending their curricula to meet new needs applies with particular force to the below-average group now being required by law to stay on at school well into adolescence. It is probably true that in the United Kingdom, the last two years of the secondary modern school have, on the whole, provided a curriculum which was designed in a previous generation for a very much more able, selected group of grammar or high-school children who were destined for a governing or managing role in the future. To some extent this situation may have been brought about by social envy, in that previously uneducated classes in the population have demanded the same kind of education as the other classes, with the result that more and more children are being exposed to a form of education which was not designed for them and for which they are not suited. It seems likely that the United Kingdom is not alone in having this particular educational problem to resolve.

It is our impression that in the Soviet Union there has been a different conception of the extension of education, which has followed there more a system of compulsory part-time education, combined with vocational training and employment. This concept needs a great deal more study in countries that have hitherto been pursuing the ideal of an academic type of education, compulsory for everybody.

The extension of school education further into late adolescence and young adulthood in many parts of the world has sometimes been attacked on the grounds that it projects an upper-class attitude onto sections of the population that have not got the necessary background. An educational psychologist described some of the different educational policies that are being followed in various countries. In Sweden, for example, students who have elected to enter those sections of the high schools that do not undertake an academic programme study more technical subjects, and arrangements are made for them to work part-time in relevant jobs for which they receive payment. They are thus able to gain more insight into what they will be doing after leaving school. The same idea has been pursued from another angle in a number of countries in which certain classes of juvenile technological employees spend part of the working week in a school provided by the employers, in order to study general educational as well as basic technological subjects. At a higher academic level, in the United Kingdom for example, so-called sandwich courses are popular, in which students spend alternate periods at university or technical college and at work.

Some of the difficulties in advancing more technical types of education at school level come from politically based opposition. Countries vary widely in this respect: in some places where the concept of school is firmly tied to an academic programme it is often found that trade unions are opposed to the teaching of technical skills in school. This opposition takes the form of refusal of trade-union membership to those who have entered the trade through school rather than through the trade's own apprenticeship arrangements (these in some instances may have remained relatively unchanged since a pre-literate period). Where the community concept of school is not so academic, the converse may be found – that entry to the trade can be secured only by a specific type of technical training conducted in schools. It was stated in the Study Group that there is some anxiety in certain circles in the United States that, because of the multiplicity of technical training schools, the more academic professions are tending to suffer by the diversion of many of the best brains into technology where, in addition, the immediate financial rewards are visibly greater.

On the side of the employers there are also difficulties about the employment of juveniles on more highly skilled technical work, relating to a feared high rate of spoilage of materials and to unduly high insurance premiums.

It was argued in discussion that expectations about schools are not always realistic. For example, it is unreasonable to anticipate that a school will completely prepare the children for work, because the conditions in school cannot be made to represent working conditions without a radical change of attitude.

On the other hand, attitudes to work at school may well be carried over into the working life of the community. Much depends on what the various sections of the community are accustomed to identify as 'work'. Thus, among the lower socio-economic groups, school learning based on reading may not be identified with 'work' at all, and the admonitions of teachers to children to devote their energies conscientiously to book learning may make little impression. Children can hardly be expected to value reading as an accomplishment when they come from homes where reading is derided. To add to the confusion, it is often considered good to work at home for pocket money. This ties a monetary reward to a certain kind of effort, which the child may be quick to recognize as being the standard condition of life for the whole family. What happens in school may appear to the child to be quite remote from the realities of life.

In those cultures in which the whole family participates in work—as in a subsistence economy—the question of education takes on a very secondary role and can hardly be separated from the needs of the workers. In such circumstances, skills of reading and writing and calculation are commonly delegated to a self-selected small section of the population which carries the responsibilities of abstract education for the whole group. In such a culture the relatively much more important question of training for work has an implicit rather than an explicit part in the community's activities. Where the whole family participates in work, the training of the younger members goes on imperceptibly and the children will learn skills and derive attitudes to working from persons with whom they have strong emotional ties. This is a training atmosphere which can never be paralleled by the more formal education given in schools because, obviously, the strength of the emotional ties between children and their teachers will not be of the same order of intensity as those with their parents.

Another respect in which schools have been manifestly ill-adapted to an industrial civilization is in preparation for adulthood and parenthood. There has been generally far too little regard to differentiation of sex in preparation for adult roles. In many countries it appears that school education makes no difference between boys and girls, with the exception sometimes of minor concessions to sex roles, such as employing boys on woodwork and metalwork during the periods when the girls are learning cookery and needlework. In either instance educational objections can be made to the teaching of such subjects in schools, other than as part of technical education in later adolescence. It appeared to members of the Study Group that, in most countries of which we have information, the different educational needs of adolescent boys and girls, from the point of view of both presentation and content of the curriculum, have not been properly evaluated and therefore not satisfactorily provided.

It is the general view among educationists that the technical aspects of teenage education are capable of being pushed too far, to the general detriment of education; that the missing out of more cultural and more abstract aspects of education does not, in the long run, lead to the greater satisfaction of ordinary people. In communities which have neglected the cultural aspects of education and have concentrated narrowly on technological work, some observers believe that a generally low level of personal satisfaction obtains.

Some of these problems are now being highlighted in communities that are proceeding to extend the period of compulsory education. In the United Kingdom, for example, for over seventy years compulsory schooling was for a nine-year period, from age five to age fourteen. This was extended by one year in 1948 to a school-leaving age of fifteen, as an intermediate step towards the goal of compulsory schooling for all to age sixteen. The difficulties encountered in implementing this first additional year gave rise to questions about the wisdom of proceeding further; finally, in 1963 a decision was taken to raise the school-leaving age to sixteen in 1970. The problems involved are not merely those of altering the flow of juveniles into industry and of training 10 per cent more teachers, though clearly these are major economic and educational factors to be considered. In 1948 the schools that had hitherto offered a non-academic type of curriculum designed to finish when their pupils were fourteen years of age were abruptly faced with the need to arrange a further year's course for which they had no practicable alternative but to borrow from existing grammar or high-school curricula. Thus both teachers and children were set an unfamiliar task, and the children were given no particular incentive such as might be supplied by school-leaving examinations. The Study Group concluded that, until a new philosophy of universal education is worked out, it may not be advantageous to increase the gap between children and the lives they will live after leaving school, in those cases in which they are not being prepared for any more academic types of interest or pursuit. It may be that the United Kingdom plan to raise the school-leaving age in two separated steps of one year has proved on the whole disadvantageous, because it has required less reshaping of the whole curriculum and has enabled the attempt to be made without radical rethinking of the whole educational aim.

Compulsory universal education until the age of sixteen or more is a great social ideal, which is tending to be adopted more and more in countries newly brought into contact with modern industrial and technological societies. But in those cultures in which education has hitherto reached only a minority of the community, there is a risk that compulsory universal primary education may do considerable violence to existing cultural attitudes, especially where education appears to the people to be an ideal imported from elsewhere. In such a case the result may be the wholesale adoption of attitudes derived from the alien school materials that it was necessary to borrow, which may have nothing to do with the indigenous culture. The Study Group agreed that the best outcome is attainable only where compulsory school attendance is recognized by both the children and the adults concerned as not only to be rooted in the familiar cultural attitudes but to have a direct bearing on the life in the future of the individual child.

An industrial psychologist summed up this discussion with the remark that nearly all schooling differs from most work in the community in one major respect: that school is essentially individual-centred, whereas work is almost always task-centred. Children are inadequately prepared by school for the changes in role and in perceptions that are involved in passing from the one to the other. On the whole, schools tend to be better at imparting information, necessary though this is, than at developing a sense of responsibility for citizenship in the children. Schools differ considerably among themselves in the extent to which their practices may be regarded as child-centred or idea-centred.

THE TRANSITION FROM ADOLESCENCE TO ADULTHOOD

Just as in very many countries the schools are not offering the type of education that, for the majority of the population, will lead them on smoothly and with due preparation into life as young adults, so the adolescent upon his entry into industrial employment is not often offered a role which he can perceive as capable of taking him into full adult life. An exception to this is to be found among that minority of the population for whom a recognized apprenticeship leads into a highly skilled occupation. Thus it is of considerable significance that the major problems of behaviour are found predominantly among the less skilled youth.

It is of great social interest that the personalities who become teenage idols tend to show qualities very different from those of the ideal figures of adults. Many of the former are glorified reflections of the teenagers themselves, their qualities being sometimes partially determined by a degree of rejection of adult values. This may be a problem of teenage identity-formation and lack of identification with adult values, and may indicate that society today is failing youth in certain respects. The Study Group was impressed by the great need to reconsider the nature and form of secondary education in relation to the values of society, and especially to the work of the older adolescent, and the kind of role that should be developed for him. One would not expect a revision of school programmes to resolve all these difficulties, not least because one of the most important sources of tension between youth and society as a whole is a particular quality of attitude among adults, which finds the behaviour of youth disturbing and may amount to quite a serious mental health problem in adults. At an anecdotal level, an educational psychologist in the Study Group related an incident at an international conference in Germany, at which there was a discussion of 'the terrible behaviour of the youth of today'. After a number of people had offered explanations, an old German lady whispered, 'I think it's just that they've got bad memories'.

It can hardly be doubted that in all modern urban industrial societies there is a complexity of relationship between school and the work that adolescents will do after leaving school. When intercultural comparisons are made, there is the additional complication that work carries a different meaning in different cultures, so that the whole idea of school and its role in society may be different also. A standard, though not universal, educational view in Europe would be that the school is part of the culture, that it should reflect cultural attitudes but not intrude into the culture in any forceful way. Thus it would be normal for the school to play some part in preparing children for an industrial life, where the community had a markedly industrial bias, and for an agricultural life where the latter was appropriate. Thus in the United Kingdom schoolchildren in agricultural areas get certain periods off when the agricultural work is at a certain phase, to help, for example, in gathering a local fruit crop. These periods do not always coincide with the school holidays determined by the needs of the industrial population, and local adjustments have to be made.

In other countries, and especially in those that are faced with the problem of large immigrant groups in processes of acculturation, the school may be used deliberately by society as a cultural instrument, and in this respect, with the full knowledge of community leaders, would intrude quite forcibly into the variegated cultural pattern of the whole society.

When the behaviour of youth differs to a significant extent from the expectations of the adults in the community it is often not difficult to divide the consequent adult attitudes into two main groups: first, those who think that the young are 'just being kids' and will settle down later, an attitude that could be covered by the generic term 'immaturity'; and those who think that the behaviour is a phenomenon of a disturbance of relationships.

The Study Group was divided in its attitude. Some members doubted whether youth behaviour problems could be completely dismissed, in the words of the old German lady quoted above, as a matter of bad memory. They thought that the rejection of adult values by members of adolescent gangs might represent a partial block in identification, in some cases amounting to an outright rejection based on indifference rather than hostility. In the case of such young people it was argued that their moral standards had not become dependent upon internalized parent figures, but had been acquired from symbols of the peer group.

This latter attitude has been well expressed in the American play *Blue Denim*, in which two youngsters drift through various sexual activities, pregnancy, abortion, etc., not from viciousness or delinquency but more from lack of parental interest and guidance. A major point of the play is that these difficulties need not have happened, because it is shown that parental sympathy can be mobilized when the nature of the problem has been made clear. According to this second view, therefore, the basic problem is that of a defect of relationship, or at least of communication, between the two generations.

The Study Group did not resolve the differences between these two attitudes, but it was agreed that the difference was more apparent than real in that what one party was referring to as a serious degree of indifference on the part of youth was regarded by the other as one aspect of a complex situation which was, at worst, ambivalent.

The anxiety felt by one generation about the behaviour of the next has on occasion been crystallized into statements to the effect that there is a tendency for a high peak of delinquency to occur in the second generation of immigrant groups. On the other hand, in the only numerical study that has been brought to our notice, Sellin (652) compared delinquency figures for first- and second-generation immigrant groups respectively in New York State and elsewhere, and found no conclusive evidence of an increase in delinquency in the second generation. A psychiatrist commented in the Study Group that the essential factor in this connexion is not migration *per se* but the amount of cultural dislocation and shattering of previous norms of behaviour that occurs. A study in the state of New Jersey showed that 60 per cent of delinquency was to be found among the immigrants from rural Southern States of the United States, who formed only 10 per cent or so of the population of the state.

In the United Kingdom, the recent influx of West Indians has tended to bring out into the open some latent anxieties about the behaviour of immigrant groups. Rumours and reports about delinquent behaviour, particularly of the children of West Indian immigrants, have tended to circulate whenever the group has become big enough in any community to be identifiable as a minority. Thus any untoward happening which previously might have passed unnoticed has immediately been focused in public attention and often ascribed to West Indians. Rumour has sometimes had it that the police have issued statements to the effect that they are on the look-out for young West Indians. This kind of rumour is rarely, if ever, substantiated, but the persistence of such untrue reports would indicate that the attention of both public and police does tend to become focused on the delinquent

49

behaviour of second-generation immigrants, irrespective of the actual incidents.

An anthropologist drew the Study Group's attention to an interesting difference between the United States and Australia in recent years, in respect of those teenage gangs that are character-ized by wearing a special group uniform, with some transvestite features. In the United States these gangs tend to be drawn from ethnic minority groups, and these are naturally often immigrants, for example, Mexicans in California, or Puerto Ricans in New York. In contrast, in Australia, the youngsters forming the similar teenage gangs, known as Widgies and Bodgies, come from British stock. The Australian population is more homogeneous than that of the United States and there are no comparable ethnic minority groups in the second generation. But the youngsters in the gangs tend to be in blind-alley jobs (juvenile employment that does not lead to a related adult trade). The generalization might be made that groups of young people who are inadequately educated and who do not have satisfying work prospects may tend to be driven back into themselves and to develop a way of life of their own. The fact of belonging to a minority group would increase the difficulty of getting jobs or adequate technical training. It was stated that in South American countries, although there were clearly identifiable minorities of Italian immigrants, social problems did not develop comparable with those of Italians in the eastern United States. It was suggested that this might be because the second-generation Italian immigrants in South America are not exposed to such wide cultural and lang-uage differences as are those in the United States, and also because they are more quickly and more completely accepted by the host society.

Thus the Study Group concluded that the problem of the late teenager moving from school and technical college into work is complex, and tends to be exacerbated by other related problems, such as movement from a childhood spent in pre-industrial surroundings into an industrial community. A psychiatrist re-marked that in the Netherlands there has been a controversy in regard to the role of university students in society. One view is that from early in their university career students should enter as far as possible into the life of the wider society; the other is that, for perhaps as much as three years, the students should live in a university enclave, taking very little part in the life of society as a whole; that their role as students should be clearly defined and distinguished from that of other members of the community. Echoes of this controversy are found in other countries, for example in the United Kingdom, between those who prefer the more segregated and strictly residential atmosphere of Oxford and Cambridge and those who favour universities in which the students are much more in touch with the life of the surrounding district.

Morris summed up the situation in a working paper by drawing attention to the many tensions that may result from failure in home, school, and college to make proper provision for helping adolescents to deal with the conflicts ensuing from the prolongation of social immaturity after the onset of physical sex maturity. He noted:

'(i) The dissatisfaction of many teenagers with prolonged schooling and their lack of abiding interest in things learned in school. (Their attempts – not all ineffective or antisocial by any means – to create their own culture and roles in the social vacuum they encounter after school form a related yet different and wider issue.)

(ii) The relatively large number of mental health "problems" thrown up in school, college, and work – not as estimated simply by official figures for maladjustment, serious mental illness, or crime, but as known personally to teachers, parents, etc.

(iii) The relative lack of maturity of large numbers of university and college students, both intellectually and emotionally.

(iv) The relatively low morale of the teaching profession, which tends to be preoccupied with status, pay, and internal or external scapegoating.'

ADAPTATION AND CHANGE

Much of the discussion on the so-called behaviour problems or delinquency of youth has a bearing on the question of adaptability to change. The concept of adaptability deserves further study, especially in regard to those situations in which the natural aggression or aggressiveness of the individual is loaded with a negative or hostile feeling. (Strictly speaking, aggression is a neutral word meaning, literally, movement towards.)

Observation of child development shows that when the outward-directed impulses of babies become organized into action they can be charged with both positive and negative affective values. According to a dynamic view of emotional development, the modification of the child's instinctual drives that takes place during the character-formation processes of early infancy tends to attach a mainly positive affective value to the instinct-modifying influences. In this way the child is released from bondage to the primitive instinct-satisfaction drives, and is free to deploy his intellectual capacity and motor skills in the real-life situation.

No less significant for the future development of the child is the positive affective value that becomes attached to the actual undergoing of change and of new experiences. Where change is presented favourably to the child, this positive attitude towards it may remain in the form of a flexibility of personality that enables the child not only easily to embrace new developments but to welcome them and seek them.

Thus, strictly speaking, it might be argued that the child does not so much adapt to change as assimilate changing processes within his own personality. Expressed simply, the toddler who learns to control bladder and bowels is in many respects not the the same child as when he was wet and dirty. This is not a question of a child merely picking up a new skill, while remaining essentially the same child. On the contrary, the developing value system of the child has undergone a radical change; never again will life for that child be as it was before he became clean. He has assimilated a major change in that his earlier values have been supplemented by more adult ones.

The above very brief reference to dynamic theory broaches a subject of enormous complexity which it is not possible to attempt to deal with at length in the current volume. Wherever a child is growing up in a family these dynamic processes of assimilation of change are affecting every member of the family circle, though in different degrees according to involvement. Thus not only does the toilet-trained toddler become a changed person by the very fact of his new-found cleanliness but his mother becomes a different person also, and other relatives change, too, in different degrees. This proposition becomes self-evident when one compares the parents and their grown-up child with the same trio during the child's early infancy.

When the whole family, together with other families, is caught up in wider processes of social change, this adds a further dimension of change to be assimilated, collectively and individually. The successful accomplishment of social and family change requires a quality of flexibility of personality in the parents as much as in the children. This concept of flexibility needs considerable qualification for use in mental health thinking in this context. In order to convey the notion of continuity and purpose, flexibility needs to be combined with some quality like resilience. In ordinary English usage, flexibility conveys an idea of something that can be bent at will, or even swayed by the wind, so that this term needs correction by the addition of the idea of the presence of inherent compensating tendencies – elasticity rather than plasticity. On the whole, flexibility calls to mind an 'other-directed' response, in contrast to the 'self-directed' response which is implied by the term resilience. The notions of self-direction and self-initiation should be introduced into the concept.

A further consideration is that change and adaptability, as applied to childhood, are not processes restricted to the earliest years. The view that the first five years of a child's life are vital is not strictly antithetical to the view that major significant changes continue to be possible to a late age. A midway position seems more consonant with fact – that the individual remains capable of change and adaptation for most of life and continues to be vulnerable to various kinds of trauma. But perhaps the curve of adaptation, if it may be expressed in such terms, starts from a low point in early infancy, rises steeply during childhood to a plateau at the end of adolescence, from which it slowly declines to a low level in old age. It is logical to suppose that the degree of satisfaction that the individual finds in the process of changing may determine to a large extent the speed and smoothness of the process, which in turn may be influenced by the actual effects on the personality brought about by changing. As remarked above, it is perhaps more accurate to think in terms of assimilation of change than in terms of adaptation.

The current prevailing psychological view is that instinct is not an entity but is composed of polymorphic tendencies which might find expression in one or more of a number of channels. This view makes the concept of adaptability more comprehensible, especially when the possibility of a latent as distinct from an absent function is taken into account. Thus the term latency might be applied to the situation in which energy is potentially there, available for dispersion through certain channels, and the more varied these channels the more potentially adaptable the individual.

It should be noted that the term flexibility, as applied to the functions of the central nervous system, implies a constitutional element. This concept was first formulated by Gross and developed by Heymans and Wiersma as 'secondary function'. Later neurological research has confirmed the existence of a constitutional factor. Thus behavioural adaptability may to some extent depend on this constitutional flexibility.

The relationship between adaptability and concepts of basic security and anxiety is complex. One dynamic view is that adaptability depends to a large extent on the satisfaction that the individual gains in the process of changing, a satisfaction that is presumably determined partly constitutionally and partly by experiences in early childhood. It is axiomatic that the individual does not gain positive satisfaction in changing unless there is considerable satisfaction also in existing conditions, though there may be relief from discomfort in change from an unsatisfactory *status quo*. Partly for this reason, anxiety is antagonistic to adaptability. If anxiety is aroused by lack of instinctual satisfaction in existing circumstances and by the frustration of impulse, the impulse to escape from unsatisfactory conditions may be weak or non-existent, especially if the individual has had no experience of more positive satisfaction. Thus strong anxiety may well tend to promote activity to restore the *status quo*, or at least to increase the search for the satisfaction to be found in the present. On the other hand, a minor degree of instinct frustration and consequent anxiety is likely to provide the main motive for the individual to seek change.

Which direction the activity aroused by anxiety will take may depend both on the degree of anxiety and on the threshold level of the individual at which mounting anxiety ceases to promote adaptive behaviour and, instead, begins to inhibit adaptation in favour of *status quo*-seeking behaviour. In practical mental health terms, then, a primary objective is to foster the ability of individuals to live with their anxiety and to raise the threshold level above which anxiety tends to paralyse adaptive behaviour.

In 'Mental Health and Value Systems' (41) the question of adaptability was considered from the point of view of identity formation, in terms of three postulated qualities of identity – flexibility, coherence, and consistency. According to this approach the *flexibility* of the identity formation is part of a *coherent* pattern so that, although adaptable, the individual remains recognizable and *consistent* with his past and the future.

On the question of adaptation to changing conditions in society and the implications for family life, the generalization is worth consideration that, where the cultural pattern is changing, the people tend to gain major satisfaction from engaging in change, but where the culture is static or on the defensive, the major satisfactions are found in maintaining the *status quo*. In the latter case change may be experienced as a threat. Thus if a previously rural population, which had lived for several generations in a subsistence economy or dependently in a tribal culture,

55

were moved suddenly to an industrial area and expected to fend for itself there in a *laissez-faire* economy, the change might appear as an overwhelming threat to the majority of the population, and might inhibit the collective adaptive behaviour to such an extent that social disorganization could result. The practical outcome would be the creation of slum conditions of life in which the people lived in great poverty. The situation of a previously well-adjusted rural community translated to a newly created slum on the outskirts of an industrial city is grim indeed. A vicious circle is almost certain to arise – the lack of satisfactions in the new life leads to frustrations that are expressed in hostilities both within the family and towards the rest of society, which decrease still further the satisfactions. The children born and reared in the slum derive their early attitudes from the atmosphere it has engendered, and unless they mix with other, more fortunately placed, children in the primary school it may not be until later in adolescence that the values of the community at large begin to impinge on them and add to the total picture of maladjustment. This social question is one of very great importance to those concerned in mental health action.

On the other hand, even in cases in which there has been an unbroken agricultural tradition and a subsistence economy, provided that their major instinctual needs continue to be met without undue stress, and also provided that the culture as a whole is not visibly threatened with extinction and that the most important relationship systems are not breaking down, there seems no reason why people should not be able to make a quick and smooth transition to a modern industrial pattern of living. This has, indeed, been the experience in some parts of the world. An anthropologist drew attention to the frequently demonstrated fact that it is often not the immigrant parents but their children who suffer most from transplantation. Where migration has been planned and where they have enough integrative capacity to maintain a minimum degree of cultural continuity, individual adults are able to make drastic changes, not only once but even perhaps three or four times in a lifetime. But children who have to grow up in a new community, learn to mix with children with far different family traditions, and go to school, are more liable to show signs of stress. Moreover, the community rarely knows how to give help to the parents so that they can make their children's acculturation less hazardous.

A unique feature of the rapidly changing conditions now prevalent in much of the world is that it is almost standard for parents to be unable effectively to help their children with the changes which have to be assimilated. This is not a difficulty that is restricted to people being translated from place to place. It might be said that the one certain thing in family life today is that the young children, when they grow up, will have to live in a world that is very different from the current world and that the nature of the difference cannot be predicted with confidence.

It is clearly a mental health concern to see what can be done by educational methods to develop flexibility and capacity to assimilate change, however unpredictable and unknown. An educational psychologist considered that the problem of education for flexibility should be seen primarily in terms of basic personality formation and security; that capacity for flexibility in response to change is related to the freedom of outgoing tendencies where there is no disabling anxiety. Of first importance, therefore, is the creation of an environment for children in which they can develop in security; but this is no more than introductory to the whole question of what children should learn and how they should learn it.

The Study Group thought that the emphasis should be put on working with the child towards creating an understanding that all learning is a personal achievement; that it is very much more than merely taking over someone else's results. The appropriation of experience through personal activity, whether by carrying out an experiment for oneself, or making a discovery, or by doing the same thing in imagination, contributes essentially to the development of the individual's capacity to handle experience in a wide variety of ways. We have referred above to the assimilation of change by the baby, a process that makes not only the child, but the whole family, into different people. Something of the same situation exists in school and it may be asked whether in most schools sufficient change is allowed for in pupil–teacher relations as the former turn into different people.

How these changes can be initiated early in the educational process is very much tied up with what styles of relationship exist between children and teachers, and with how teachers view their responsibilities. So many teachers conceive of their essential function as the transmission of what are known as facts, forgetting that facts are, as it were, fossilized forms of acts. If a generalization is permissible, in the educational sphere there is a need to make changes in the direction of securing more flexibility, even at quite a late stage in education. In the selection of education students, for example, it is important to look for the capacity not only to acquire professional skills but to be critical of such skills, and to appraise the individual's reasons for taking up teaching; and, in teacher-training, to promote the ability to evaluate what can be done with the skills that are acquired. Teachers in general need to come to a clearer idea of what it is they want to do with children.

SOME STRESS PHENOMENA IN MODERN SOCIETY

Signs of stress in modern society are many and vary more with cultural attitudes than with the actual stresses encountered. This is particularly true of such widespread stress phenomena at alcoholism, drug addiction, and disorders of sexual conduct, to the extent that quantitative cross-cultural comparisons cannot be safely made in these respects.

The Study Group thought that more suitable fields for cross-cultural study in contemporary urban and industrialized society could be found in the processes of transition from youth to adulthood, and in the relative positions of men and women in society. All over the world, in the more developed countries, the middle teenage period appears to be characterized by group behaviour which causes the adults in the society a great deal of anxiety.

Another neglected field is that of grief and mourning. Universally, at all levels of civilization, societies that have a settled tradition have well-established social institutions and ceremonies to deal with tragedy and bereavement, and they form an essential part of the adjustment of the bereaved individual to the new situation. In a rapidly changing and developing society, such ceremonies may be lost or become severely modified, with the result that the individual is left to deal with his grief by himself, without the help of a familiar framework. As Bowlby's studies of grief in infancy (653, 654, 655) have suggested, a primary aspect of the individual's reaction to bereavement is rage (which may go on to a state of apathy), and it is a logical inference that much of funeral ritual is concerned with the control of these feelings. Bereavement may therefore constitute a serious mental health problem in changing societies, and also an interdisciplinary problem of considerable religious and social significance.

In the United States at the present time, for example, there appears to be almost a widespread conspiracy to keep the facts of death from children. It is not uncommon for town-dwelling American children to reach quite an advanced age before being confronted with the concrete phenomenon of death – though in the world of cinema and television fantasy death is a commonplace. On the other hand, funeral rituals have proliferated in the States, among certain sections of the population, to a very remarkable degree. Interestingly, many of these rituals serve to predicate the denial of death, such as the make-up of the deceased person, lying in an open or glass-lidded coffin. The tremendous fuss and display surrounding interment can hardly be due merely to morticians' keen business methods; they must correspond to a need.

The multidisciplinary involvement in problems of bereavement was well illustrated after the great fire in Boston, where it was found that many of the bereaved presented acute depressive conditions which required a working through of mourning and guilt associated with the disaster. The Study Group noted that these and other disaster situations present unique opportunities for interdisciplinary study. The example cited, of a group of people in an acute state of mourning, would enable much to be learned about the differences between normal and pathological mourning.

STRESS AND VULNERABILITY IN CHILDREN

In a working paper, Skard posed the question of which stresses and conflicts affect the greatest number of children in a particular culture. In other words, are those stress situations which result in difficulties specific to the children concerned in each case; or are virtually all children exposed to stresses but only a few develop symptoms? If the latter, what governs the outcome – whether children develop stress phenomena, or go through unharmed, or perhaps emerge strengthened for further development? She quoted a case of a Norwegian boy, one of a group of eighteen presumably normal children, whose development was followed up to eight years of age:

'Tom was the younger of two siblings, only eleven months younger than his sister. This pregnancy was unwanted, the mother even wanted abortion, but was forbidden to go through with it by the father. The mother disliked the care of babies. Tom was breast-fed for eight days, bottle-fed for four to five months, then fed by cup and spoon, always at fixed times of the day. From the age of about four months until about eight months Tom was away from the parents and lived with the maternal grandparents, then came back to the parents again. From the age of one year onwards, he was being toilet-trained and severely punished for accidents. He was not "clean and dry" until he was more than three years old. From the age of two he was sent daily to play under supervision in the park. But he soon started wandering all over the town, frequently not coming home until night. The father was very severe and spanked Tom from the time he was very small, and so hard that at times the mother was afraid that his kidneys might be damaged. Between the ages of five and seven years Tom was judged by all observers to be one of the best-adjusted and healthiest children of our sample.'

The unsolved question is: how did Tom manage to cope with all these difficulties without suffering apparent harm?

Skard raises the problem of whether there are *generally critical* periods when children are more vulnerable to conflict-forming influences, or whether children may be vulnerable to different kinds of special stress at different stages of development. She further suggests that it may be possible to apply to psychological development the principle of vulnerability that holds in the case of somatic development, that a structure or function in a state of particularly rapid growth is modifiable to a relatively high degree. From this it might be inferred that there are both generally critical periods of rapid development, when children are vulnerable to conflict-forming influences, and specific stages at which the individual child is susceptible and which relate to the individual pattern of development.

Again, children at different age levels may show various forms of reaction to stress and have different ways of coping with difficulties. The increased intellectual potential of the child of between eight and eleven years of age, for example, provides a better tool for working on problems than that of younger children. On the other hand, the disturbances of emotional equilibrium that may be characteristic of some children at puberty can make an adolescent more vulnerable to certain kinds of stress.

In a working paper quoted extensively elsewhere in this Report, Soddy made a comparison between a child brought up in a unique relationship with a single mother-figure and one brought up as a member of a family group of perhaps a dozen people. He suggests that the respective vulnerabilities of these two children might be at quite different levels. For example, under the age of two years or so the child with a single mother-figure would almost certainly be vulnerable to the absence of his mother, but it might matter comparatively little where the child was, or what his mother actually did with him. The child in a large family group, in contrast, would be more likely to be vulnerable to change of circumstances and style of living, but perhaps not so much to the presence or absence of a particular individual. This is only one of many aspects of vulnerability that might be considered.

THE PROBLEM OF ANXIETY

The perennial problem in this area is that of anxiety, in both its individual and its group aspects. Though anxiety is a universal phenomenon, its manifestations are extremely diverse. In a settled agricultural community with a traditional style of life one would anticipate that anxiety, such as it may be, would be canalized mainly on to climate, rainfall, pests, and so on. In a rapidly developing industrial society, apart from worries about work and learning new things and generally strange conditions, there is also likely to be a high index of anxiety over family relationships and the ability of the individual to be successful in social life; though there would be wide variations in the degree to which anxiety became consciously explicit (which would to a great extent depend on the cultural situation). That the admission of anxiety to consciousness can reach quite a high degree of sophistication was shown by a recent United States study on the evaluation of anxiety, reported by Ewalt in a working paper:

'What people say: A scientifically selected national sample was interviewed by a team of professionally trained interviewers. The purpose was to determine the sources of happiness and satisfaction and the sources of worry and unhappiness among our people, and the schedules were so constructed that we could know much about the kind of people giving the answers. We found that one person in four said he had at some time worried so much that he feared a "nervous breakdown" but only one in seven actually sought help. Identifying problems as psychological in origin was associated with the younger age group, the better educated, and those of higher income. People tended to find happiness in their families and their work and they tended to be distressed by family problems, economic worries, and in the older group by worry over health.'

The most prevalent forms of anxiety to be found in highly

developed industrial communities that have been undergoing processes of social change for some generations may be seen in the field of religion, where generally traditional items of faith tend to be questioned and new concepts of the relationship between God and man are constantly being propounded by small religious movements. One of these, though perhaps of not more than a quasi-religious character, is the cultivation of peace of mind and relaxation, the application of some of the practices of Yoga without a grasp of the underlying attitudes and principles. In a more psychological sphere can be found the modern concern with introspection which has led to existentialist concepts of God.

A clergyman described some of the recent new sources of religious anxiety that have been opened up by the imminence of space travel. For example, in Judeo-Christian theology, the concept of God has grown from that of a tribal god to a god of the whole world, but hitherto only vaguely of the universe. Now the ordinary person is having to face the possibility of contact with other worlds and conceivably other universes. This is a potential source of anxiety, of the same order as the anxiety which must attend the giving up of a notion of a tribal god in order to share the divinity with a much wider group of people.

In a working paper, Pacheco e Silva reported that many examples of the proliferation of manifestations of anxiety can be found in Latin American countries which, as has been stated elsewhere, have been highly subjected to processes of rapid change in recent years. Thus even under the umbrella of Roman Catholicism one can find the widespread diffusion of primitive animism, *macumba*, *candombles*, and other rites of African or Americo-Indian origin. In times of great distress or social disorganization, many prophets, mystics, and reformers arise and start small religious movements. Folklore and folk music and dance reveal much evidence of magical thinking, belief in the malevolent powers of certain persons (*Jetaturas*), and superstitions of the most irrational character.

Biesheuvel drew attention to similar phenomena in Southern Africa, where indigenous people at a more primitive state of civilization have been brought more sharply into contact with modern industrial life, imposed by a completely alien culture that is presented to them in a relationship of superiority-inferiority. He points out that whereas traditional African societies are by no means free from anxiety – chiefly related to their poor control over the material environment, ignorance concerning natural phenomena, and belief in spiritual influences – there are also ample and institutionalized means of defence, reassurance, and catharsis.

As tribal society has broken down, although belief in spiritual agencies has not necessarily diminished, ritual practices of a defensive or abreactive nature have fallen into disuse, maybe because they could not function outside the intact tribal society, or else have been forbidden by law (e.g. trial by ordeal, ritual murder). This loss of traditional practices has occurred in a setting in which change and loss of the familiar way of life have already greatly increased anxiety. Biesheuvel wrote:

'New anxieties are also arising on the score of status needs and satisfactions. Status in traditional societies was associated with the role one was called upon to perform. Individual effort, or personal choice and qualities had very little to do with this. Conformity was the major virtue and individuality was tolerated only within particular spheres. In the new society, however, status is a measure of personal achievement. Occupational and political life has provided ample scope for the satisfaction of new personal ambitions, but the price in terms of stress has still to be assessed. It is true that, with the trend towards other-direction in personality development, conformity needs are also important. But because this type of conformity arises in response to a social system with constantly changing fads and fashions, an uppercrust of ephemeral values, and a diffuse reference group, it cannot give the assurance to be derived from conforming to a stable social order with fixed habits, based on clearcut prescriptions for conduct, and displayed by familiar people in one's immediate environment. As we have seen, Riesman considers diffuse anxiety to be a motive force in other-directed personalities.'

Biesheuvel indicated the additional stress that is imposed upon Africans who are trying to adjust to a rapidly changing social order if they find that both custom and law discriminate between different groups. Very difficult situations may arise, leading to personality breakdown, when Africans have to function in an intermediary position, employed and supervised by Whites, but themselves directing the work of Black labourers. Such situations can be particularly severe when an African has to administer or enforce laws that are unpopular with his own people.

'There are very few comparative studies between Black and White, or between African groups living under urbanized and traditional conditions. Research is complicated by lack of knowledge concerning normal African personality development, and the manner in which effective disorder manifests itself in traditional cultures. The extent of the availability of mental health services and the frequency of referral is another complicating circumstance.

There are indications from observational, interview, and projective studies that anxiety is a common feature of the mental state of normal Africans today. There are also indications that the need to discharge this anxiety has led to an increased belief in the potency of witchcraft. In this respect African thinking has retained its culturally determined character, even after so much else in the traditional culture has disintegrated. This may be due to the fact that it is satisfying to be able to locate the source of one's distress outside the self, in an objective even though spiritual form. In this form it can be dealt with by means of time-honoured methods of an equally objective and spiritual type. The structure of African personalities, particularly where they are still partly the product of traditional upbringing, also favours this projective, extrovert response.

A number of social anthropologists have commented on the

extent to which the practice and fear of witchcraft have increased in tribal communities which are beginning to feel the impact of Western culture. Supporting evidence is also provided in a study by M. J. Field on mental disorder in rural Ghana (556), which shows that new shrines to native deities continue to be founded "in response to a search for security begun about forty years ago, concurrently with the rise of the cocoa industry. The majority of the pilgrims are healthy people who supplicate for protection against witchcraft." '

4
Population Problems

One of the greatest sources of anxiety in many parts of the world is the extraordinarily rapid rate at which world population figures are increasing. This expansion has tremendous social implications in addition to the obvious anxiety it arouses about how the increased population can be fed. Not only has the world population increased by four or five times in the last 150 years, but current trends show that the rate of increase is accelerating. Increasing density of population has led to the formation of vast new urban areas, resulting, as discussed elsewhere, in radical upheavals of patterns of social and family life. The very fact of a big population increase compels social and family change on a wide scale.

The field of interest of mental health in connexion with the population increase is wide and complex, and its rational discussion is made more difficult by the existence of various religious and ideological taboos. Because of these, it needs to be emphasized clearly that the concern of the Study Group here is with the mental health implications of the whole field of population problems. That is, we have to take into account the fact of population increase, the problems of nutrition, movement, and interpersonal relations that are implied, and the measures proposed for mitigating the effects or possibly for preventing the increase. We are concerned no less with the reasons why some people advocate measures of birth control and fertility control; and why other groups are opposed to one or both of these types of measure on religious, ideological, and/or political grounds.

The Study Group was at pains to note that, because a particular method of solving a problem might be taboo or anathema to a certain section of the population, this does not alter the fact that the problem might be a serious one, demanding a solution. It is a matter of extremely important principle that the problem be not ignored or evaded merely because of some notion of respecting the feelings of people who regard its discussion, or some aspect of its possible solution, as dangerous or taboo.

The fact is sometimes overlooked that birth control is only one of a number of measures that have been considered in relation to rapidly increasing populations; and also that this particular measure has been opposed not only on religious or moral grounds, notably by the Roman Catholic church, but also on ideological or political grounds by many nations or other groups nervous of their economic or military strength. It may be a matter of discussion as to how far it is legitimate to consider these four grounds for opposition as if they were completely separable.

Among the mental health questions involved in any attempt to control population increase may be cited, for example, the effect of attempts to modify or change the direction of the reproductive behaviour of people of different cultures and with different levels of social and political aspiration. There may be many indirect effects, over a wide range, from anxiety about military supremacy, on the one hand, to worry about the sexual behaviour of the young and concern about what would happen to attitudes to virginity if birth-control techniques were to become popularized and freely available, on the other. To divert the attention now given to birth control to fertility control might resolve some of the existing tensions in relation to current taboos, e.g. certain codes of moral behaviour that have developed defensively, but it could not provide a complete answer to difficulties. Such action would probably create new areas of anxiety, not only with regard to the basis of interference with natural reproduction, but also, at a more irrational level, in terms of the possibility of harming the reproductive processes, of increasing mental deficiency, and the like.

Birth and fertility control are not the only possible ameliorative measures for problems of population increase. Better food distribution could make a notable contribution to resolving the problems, and from the point of view of mental health any change in the current world food situation would be likely to be an improvement. The present position is that some countries are spending vast sums of money in order to store surplus food (we understand that the United States alone is spending some five million dollars every year to store surplus food) while the majority of the world's population is still living below an optimum subsistence level, and an unknown proportion is living under conditions not far removed from starvation. The situation could hardly be worse in this respect and this vast human problem is of unparalleled importance. However, the redistribution of food surpluses over the world is a complex issue, involving not only problems of transport and monetary exchange, but also a radical alteration of the balance of international relationships and attitudes towards other peoples.

Another mental health aspect of the population problem which has not been studied sufficiently is the fact that whereas, with a few exceptions, a country will usually regard with satisfaction an increase in its own population, population increases in other countries will tend to be considered a threat or a disaster. We have referred above (p. xxviii) to our dislike of the term 'population explosion', perhaps the most popular current term in use in discussing these problems. 'Population explosion' is a highly evocative expression in this age of nuclear weapons, a term that puts the phenomenon in its most threatening light. One member of the Study Group remarked that it appears from the way in which the term is commonly used that a population explosion is something that happens in another country – not in one's own. As remarked above, a vast increase in population in one's own country appears with very few exceptions to be regarded with equanimity, in spite of a possible lowering in the standard of living. Apart from the doubtful example of Japan, there has been no historical example so far of a country successfully limiting its population increase for political and economic reasons. In contrast, an increase in population in another, and particularly a neighbouring country, may be interpreted as a threat, whether to national security or cultural influence, or even in many cases to the standards of living of the whole world. When the increase is very rapid, 'explosion' is the word that precisely fits the feeling.

The Study Group was concerned with what can be done about these matters from the mental health point of view. In the words of an anthropologist member, 'It is no good telling other people that they should not have children'. Yet the advocacy of population control without clarity about the unconscious as well as the conscious significance of such action may amount virtually to telling others not to have children for ego-centred reasons.

This is an area of change of attitude which requires the most careful study. The processes of bringing about change in the interests of mental health which we have discussed include the gaining of the support of the network of influence in any given community for the proposed change. Generally speaking, this can be done only with what might be termed an ideology-free vocabulary, or, in other words, by advocating change in ways that do not provoke emotionally determined resistance because of conflict with important values. On the contrary, success in changing attitudes may depend to a large extent on the degree to which it is possible to harness the positive feelings that are based on such values. No question illustrates these points more clearly than that of population control. No mental health organization can take up a definite position either in regard to birth control or in regard to fertility control without resolving the many conflicting attitudes derived from religious, ideological, and political motives. It might be possible to resolve some of the religious or moral difficulties by transferring the main attention from contraception to fertility control. When people had got used to the idea, this might meet some of the moral objections that are now raised to birth control. But if the underlying unconscious processes are not dealt with, it is equally possible that new and compelling moral objections might arise to fertility control.

In attempts to get round moral or ideological objections, ways of decelerating population growth other than fertility control are often advocated, for example, later marriage or sexual continence within marriage, but the Study Group thought that no proposals have yet come forward effectively to overcome the practical obstacles to success that arise out of the kinds of feeling that have resulted in the use of this term 'population explosion' for the felt danger of the rapid population increase in a country other than one's own. It should be noted that the current very high rates of increase are not restricted to underdeveloped countries, and although anxiety about the phenomenon is at its strongest in Western Europe and North America, the rate of population increase in the United States is among the highest in the world. When, as sometimes happens, countries with a static or falling population, or other countries with a high standard of living and a rapidly increasing population become identified as the chief protagonists of population control for other, less developed, countries in a state of rapid expansion, the reaction among the latter must inevitably defeat the objective.

RACISM, PREJUDICE, AND DISCRIMINATION

Many people today rate the problems of interrace[1] or intergroup relationships and the hostilities they evoke as second in importance to humanity, only to the threat of annihilation through nuclear warfare. These two problems are intimately connected, if only for the very obvious reason that with increased capacity for mutual destruction the threat inherent in mutual hostility becomes greater too, especially at a time when the enormous improvement in communications, combined with a great increase in population, has brought the question of intergroup relationships to the forefront of the world's attention. It would, perhaps, be cynical to say that intergroup relations have worsened generally throughout the world precisely because of the greater proximity resulting from the above factors, but there can be no doubt that

[1] The term 'race' is being employed in its current loose or colloquial usage to signify a recognizable and transmitted configuration of physical characteristics by which human beings may be grouped. In this discussion we have used the term 'racism' in preference to the more familiar 'racialism'.

the potential consequences of bad group relations are now catastrophic.

The issues of interrace and intergroup relations bring the question of prejudice and discrimination into sharp relief, and the Study Group took note of valuable research work that had been done in the period under review on defining the factors that contribute to hostile prejudice in people's attitudes (568). For example, it is now generally accepted that the 'authoritarian personality' can be defined more or less precisely and its strongly developed form is regarded by some people as a personality disorder of considerable seriousness.

The literature in this area is voluminous (569). In WFMH Introductory Cross-cultural Study No. 1 on 'Identity' (40), there is some discussion from the mental health point of view on how both positive and negative prejudice could be implanted by relating children's approved behaviour to the values of the in-group and disapproved behaviour to the out-group. This is only one of many studies attempting to tackle the difficulties and dangers that prejudice and discrimination create.

In 'Mental Health and Value Systems' (41) the point is again touched upon in advocacy of what is termed the 'principle of positivism' – that identity should be defined in positive terms and not by describing what the individual is not. This point will be elaborated below.

One of the great difficulties in this field is to find a satisfactory terminology. It has been pointed out with justification that the terms 'prejudice' and 'discrimination' are both neutral, and that it is equally possible to be prejudiced or to discriminate in favour of, as against. A French psychiatrist noted that the same difficulty is found in French: *préjugé* is an ambivalent term, and *discrimination* a mathematical term of complete neutrality. He remarked that difficulty in finding a word to express a sentiment may be due to an unconscious block because of which the sentiment cannot be fully integrated into the personality. In other words, the existence of negatively prejudiced attitudes may militate against the finding of a satisfactory definition; for unless the individual has full psychological insight, it is an important aspect of ego strength to be unprejudiced, as far as conscious awareness goes.

The psychiatrist suggested that 'prejudice against' can best be defined in terms of feelings of superiority and hostility; but as far as race attitudes are concerned the phenomena of racism are complex in that, in addition to hostility, they include the fascination of one group by another. According to this view, a racist is a man who is afraid of another group, but at the same time fascinated by the other party and in a sense 'in love' with it.

It has been said that prejudice is the father of discrimination; that where a group of people share in common a prejudice against an individual or another group, this will be the start of discriminatory action against the other party. But, as a social psychologist pointed out, the reverse is also true. Moreover, where an individual is reminded constantly by the institutions of his own society that other people are not like himself, these institutions will themselves create prejudice; or, in other words, prejudice and discrimination can constitute a vicious spiral.

The social psychologist spoke of the multidimensional nature of these questions, which include problems of mental health, of personal insecurity, and of social institutions and therefore legislation; there are also cognitive problems involved, in respect of false images or stereotypes, which no doubt similarly have a multiple causation.

The word racism is not ideal in this connexion, but none better is available. The negative attitudes that the word racism implies are, of course, not always or necessarily directed against others of a different race. They may well be aimed at people of a different religion or ethnic background, or even of a different social class within the same culture. Among the variety of attitudes shown by groups towards other groups, there are some negative attitudes of a more general and widespread nature which are not a monopoly of any one group. It is probably true that because white people have, in recent generations, tended to occupy a position of superiority in the world, they have played a more decisive part than other peoples in the development of what has been called racist attitudes. But it should not be forgotten that a racism that starts from the possession of a darker skin is potentially just as dangerous and disruptive of human relationships as one that springs from the possession of a lighter skin.

It is of profound significance in the modern world that problems of interpersonal relationships within countries can no longer be treated exclusively as purely domestic matters in which the rest of the world has no interest. This fact applies specifically to the problems of intergroup relations. It could not possibly be maintained that the problem of Algeria was exclusively a French matter, or that the questions of interrace relations in South Africa and of school integration in the United States concern only those countries. It is now fully recognized, in the case of South Africa, that each new development in the political situation has caused a ferment through Africa and Asia, and that the present struggle is being followed anxiously in every country in the world.

To maintain that there are certain issues, such as intergroup hostilities, that affect the whole world is not the same as to claim an automatic right for individuals to intervene across national boundaries because of the involvement of some principle in which they are vitally interested. Among the complex issues involved, the Study Group rates highly the absolute necessity not to impose value judgements cross-culturally, without due regard to the applicability of the judgement. An illustration can be given from the recent history of Ghana, where a large proportion of influential leaders who are not actively in support of the government have been subjected to detention for long periods. In a country with a mature democratic system and a high standard of education, such a situation would be completely incompatible with any ideal of a parliamentary democracy; however, in a country where the constitution is quite new, where the experience of an elected government is still within the first generation, where the majority of the electorate are illiterate, and where, because of geographical remoteness and lack of education, the majority are not in a position to make judgements on complex issues, the same freedom of expression and personal rights can hardly be afforded as in the more mature democracy. These are some of the factors to be taken into account before someone from another country who believes in the right of free speech and the political freedom of the individual can be justified in attempting to interfere.

One factor that appeared to the Study Group to be pertinent to the question whether intervention was justified was the degree of universality that the violated values had. If an issue or a piece of legislation in a particular country runs counter to values that are shared by much or most of the world, then the events in that country in this respect are of concern to the whole world. This may well be true where the issues involve racial superiority or inferiority, and attempts by one section of the population to keep another section in a permanently inferior condition. Such attempts would appear to repudiate values which, if not universal, are held by the majority of people all over the world.

In mental health circles it is usual to wish to combat prejudiced attitudes and discriminatory action, mainly on the grounds of the pathological effects on the personality formation of both parties, and especially of the dominant party. But there are complex practical questions in tackling problems of conflict based on race attitudes, in finding out which techniques work best in what circumstances. In a working paper, Biesheuvel advocated a three-point approach:

'(i) to encourage more rational thinking about race differences by all the means at our disposal;
(ii) to reduce the severity of economic conflict, which often exploits racial differences, by raising the productivity of all categories of labour, by removing gross inequalities in standards of living, and by providing a reasonable level of social security for all;
(iii) to remove and to prevent legal discrimination, but to tolerate some measure of customary exclusiveness in social practices.'

Biesheuvel warned against the attempt to tackle race prejudice by relying on arguments to prove to the ordinary man that some

75

of his attitudes about race have no foundation. There is a very wide gulf between scientific thinking and popular feeling in these matters. Geneticists attack the validity of the concept of race differences, pointing out that there are virtually no pure races and that people of all races have the majority of their genes in common. Thus it is not difficult to show the reality of genetic overlap in respect of biological qualities – that there are Negroes with blue eyes, that some Australian Aborigines have long, blonde hair, and so on. However scientifically convincing these arguments may be, Biesheuvel noted, when they are put to the non-scientific man in the street his reaction may be only that someone is trying to sell him something. If a scientist tells him that differences that appear to him to be obvious – as, for example, dark skin and 'crinkly' hair, which he has always called racial – have no real existence, the man in the street merely becomes distrustful of science.

In such a case it can be argued that it is far better to adopt a different approach, and to concede that it is perfectly easy to distinguish by various biological characteristics between some of the groups in question. In order to avoid a debate that is quite irrelevant in this context, about what constitutes race, it is better to press the question energetically, whether the differences between two groups are as relevant as has been traditionally thought; whether many of the differences are not purely cultural, subject to constant change, and removable by means of education.

This brought the discussion to consideration of Biesheuvel's second point: it was noted that a cultural approach to problems of inequality may be appropriate in many circumstances, but arguments along such lines will prove ineffective if they fail to take account of the highly important fact that attempts to promote race equality usually involve challenges to privileged positions. It is undeniable that in societies in which discriminatory practices are the rule there are gross social inequalities between the various groups and, as an inevitable accompaniment, strong social pressures to maintain the inequalities.

From the psychological point of view it would be sounder to

try to alleviate such situations by creating different types of social institution which tend to remove the threat, rather than by relying on educational, cultural, or biological arguments. For example, it is usually not difficult for people to appreciate that the presence of a group in the population at a lower standard of living and deficient in technical skills must necessarily be a source of weakness – economic, social, and cultural – and can never be a source of strength to the community. Moreover, the energy and force required to maintain the group in a position of permanent inferiority can only reduce the prosperity and the opportunities for constructive living of all the rest of the community. Thus, the fear of being supplanted by the underprivileged group operates most strongly in these circumstances – a fear that will arise at its strongest in a society whose members conceptualize their group differences as divisions and who cannot conceive intergroup relationships in terms other than those of superiority-inferiority. The ironical fact of this situation is that if the superior group does not admit the possibility of cooperation and integration with the inferior group, its own continued existence will be dependent on its capacity to maintain the *status quo*. If for numerical, material, or moral reasons, there should be a change in the balance of political power, the result will be the elimination of the previous ruling class – a historical fact that has been repeatedly illustrated by violent revolution, throughout history, and in recent times by events in the Belgian Congo.

The attempt to remove discrimination by legislation is usually an essential part of egalitarian movements, although the opinion is gaining ground that laws can change attitudes only indirectly, whereas attitudes can change laws directly. Class exclusiveness is one of the most enduring of social phenomena and has persisted for centuries even in the longest-established democratic countries. For example, in Great Britain where, in England at least, there has been an unbroken tradition establishing the equal rights of individual citizens by law for 750 years, the last major piece of anti-discrimination legislation is no older than 150 years. As Biesheuvel remarked in his working paper:

'One can legislate against occupational discrimination, but "love thy neighbour" can be only a moral, and not a statutory, injunction. Given time, the experience of working together on common tasks is bound to create, if not affection, then at least respect. And where there is mutual respect race antagonisms lose their dangerous potency.'

Biesheuvel's third approach, to attack discriminatory legislation wherever it occurs, is on firmer ground. Any regulation in a community which forbids a certain class of citizen to do something which other citizens regard as their right deserves the most critical scrutiny. However much this may appear to be a statement of simple social justice, it is better not to confuse the major issue by attempting at the same time to limit the right of social groups to take cooperative action in the interest of their own group. For example, the right of individuals to form a social club reserved for individuals of a certain colour of skin or some other socially recognizable distinction might be disapproved, but it cannot legitimately be challenged on grounds of discrimination, provided that membership of the club is entirely voluntary, and also provided that lack of membership does not carry with it automatic disqualification from the fullest participation in the life of the community.

The Study Group wished to emphasize that its concern with problems of racial antagonism at this stage of the discussion was not primarily because such antagonism might result from and/or cause bad mental health, but rather because bad community relations anywhere inevitably have wide repercussions. Biesheuvel summed up the position:

'Group antagonisms based on race are intractable, because they involve an awareness of biological differences which cannot be altered in the way one can alter religious affiliation by conversion, and political partisanship by propaganda.

Racial discrimination does not rest solely on prejudice and ignorance. Even when it is appreciated that most of, if not all, the differences associated with race are of cultural origin, social distance may still be maintained because of a preference for particular ways of living.

More serious is the conflict of interest that may be at the root of racial discrimination. Competition in labour markets, threats to standards of living, and the challenge to a privileged political position are all realities that underlie racial conflicts in those cases where the economic and political demarcation lines happen to coincide with those of race. This kind of conflict cannot be removed merely by exposing false beliefs and stereotyped thinking; but when placed in its proper perspective, race conflict, in so far as it is economic in origin, becomes amenable to the conventional means employed for the resolution of politico-economic differences in general. Even though this may not reduce the acuteness of these differences, it ensures that they will be seen in a rational light, with fewer reflections on human dignity and fewer emotionally tinged shadows.'

In his working paper on diminution of prejudice, Rees made an analogy between (hostile) prejudice and an endemic disease, and wondered whether we might not attempt to eliminate prejudice by building up 'antibodies' in children. Rees stated:

'Most people have some kind of understanding of malaria, which is tiresome, dangerous, damaging to health, and has always been recognized, correctly, as a killer disease. Few people think of prejudice as being similarly a killer disease, which needs to be diminished, if it cannot in fact be entirely eradicated. Prejudice was responsible for some six million deaths in central Europe, as the Eichmann trial has recently reminded us. It has killed a very large number on the India-Pakistan borders; and it is still killing people in a dozen or more countries. It is seriously damaging the lives and efficiency and "quality of living" of people in most countries of the world.

. . . Prejudice is not merely a killer. It is an endemic disease, which has always been present from the earliest days of history. It is epidemic, in that it flares up pretty constantly,

79

usually when a minority group in the general population reaches a certain size – it has sometimes been thought to be about 15 per cent of the total group, in a school, a community, or a nation.'

This arresting analogy imparts a great sense of urgency which the subject clearly deserves, but there is a danger that its dramatic quality will lead to the analogy being pressed too far. At a psychological level, prejudice is not a matter of the invasion of the psyche by dangerously contagious concepts which do not normally exist in the human mind, but rather a disturbance of the balance of normal thought-processes.

In a working paper, Mead remarked:

'We should propose a programme which would emphasize research and action in the development of a positive sense of personal, family, community, and national identity. We should ask, not, *what makes a person prejudiced against members of other groups?*, but, *what kind of group membership needs no derogation of others in order to maintain itself?* What kind of definition of being male or female, Caucasian, Negroid, or Mongoloid, citizen of one national state rather than another, is free of any trace of lowering another group in order to define one's own? As long as male means *not* female, Caucasian means *not* coloured, Jewish means *not* Christian, prejudice is the invariable accompaniment of contented group membership.

As a preface, to avoid the traditional exclusive position, it is necessary to substitute phrasing such as:

"There are two sexes, and I am a female"
"There are several large racial groups; I am a Caucasian"
"There are many nations; I am a Pole, or an American, or a Thai."

When one's own group is stated as one among others, the need to derogate and depreciate as part of maintaining one's own identity vanishes. A great deal of work has been done in studying the way in which prejudice grows and flourishes, the way in which special interest groups exploit it for their own ends, and the way in which it becomes a festering point in the personalities of the mentally unbalanced. We now need – as a counterbalance – an equal amount of attention paid to the ways in which a society, a community, or a family can achieve and structure group membership positively.'

Rees proposed that important investigations be made into prejudice formation on the following lines:

(i) careful sampling studies to gain evidence about the age at which negatively prejudiced attitudes begin to appear in children;
(ii) the degree of correspondence between parental attitudes and the prejudices expressed by young children;
(iii) the effect on children of parental change of attitude through education;
(iv) the effect on parents' attitudes of factual information assimilated by the children at school.

Rees was also concerned with the effect of children's literature, films, television, and broadcasting. It has been suggested, for example, that stories like 'Little Black Sambo' and 'Epaminondas' tend to promote prejudiced attitudes. To what extent would it be possible to combat negative prejudice by similar techniques?

THE PSYCHODYNAMICS OF SEGREGATION

In a working paper Levy described a research project in the Psychiatric Department of the Tulane Medical School, New Orleans, Louisiana, which had the object of ascertaining the various influences bearing on a given white individual that determined his attitude towards the segregation of Negroes in the State. The first sample studied was composed of native-born Louisianians recruited from the personnel files of Tulane University; the second sample was taken from an industry; and third and fourth samples were planned from small urban and rural areas respectively.

The term 'segregation' was related to the views of 'one who supports the notion that the races should not mingle, in terms of marriage, social hierarchy, fraternization, etc., but rather must be kept isolated'. 'Desegregation' was related to the views of 'one who wishes to be free of any law, provision, or practice requiring isolation of a particular race in separate units, especially in education or the military'. Varying degrees of emotional investment in the attitude expressed, and in the activity employed in furthering the attitude, were also defined.

During a guided informal interview, the interviewer made sure that a range of topics under seven major headings was covered. (The subject was told that the material would be used only for scientific purposes, and that his identity would be completely protected.)

(i) Travel: the subject's experience of travel in other states of and outside the United States, differentiating pleasure trips from visits long enough to know 'the people'. Military experience. Awareness of differences found in other places in attitudes towards Negroes. Influence of travel on own attitudes and regional or national loyalties.

(ii) Contemporary influences on the subject's attitudes: i.e. family, friends, community leaders, newspapers. Attitude to interference from non-Southerners. Contemporary contact with Negroes at work or in the home (domestic, etc.). Special study of influence of public personalities on the subject, of crowd atmospheres; his attendance at meetings on segregation topics, and membership of special political groups related to the issue. His identification – urban or rural.

(iii) School: teachers' attitudes, and any significant teacher with a particular influence. Books, school-books, TV, movies, plays, etc.

(iv) Teaching in childhood: concerning Negroes, and family attitudes, including subject's estimate of the most important influence. Childhood experiences with Negro children and adults, including servants, play, other children's experiences.

First awareness of colour difference and young childhood theories about differences. Concept of differences, early fears and dreams of Negroes, instances of trauma.

(v) Religion: subject's concept of religious teaching about Negroes; influence of Sunday school and minister's attitude.

(vi) Doubts, anxieties, conscience: self-doubts and guilt about attitudes, changes and crises. Statement of how segregation, if successful, would affect Whites in general. What subject thinks will really happen (interviewer records prejudices – *but not* direct questioning). Anxiety about social, sexual, economic, educational, and other aspects. Symptoms: dreams, sleep, headaches, etc.

(vii) Subject's general appearance, and interaction between interviewer and subject.

Following the interview the subject was asked to check on a list his impression of the interviewer's attitude towards segregation versus desegregation. In the main, the subject believed that the interviewer was in agreement with him. At the end of the interview the subject was placed in a particular category and rated on a four-point scale: extreme, marked, moderate, mild.

Levy reported that, to the time of writing, the subjects had been very cooperative indeed, very interested in telling their viewpoints and in taking part in a 'scientific project'. It was hoped that the application of a case-study method would enable the psychodynamics of attitude development to be formulated, and provide a check on existing psychological theories.

In concluding this discussion, the Study Group reiterated its conviction that the best role of the Federation in this and similar controversial areas is the positive illumination of the psycho-social factors involved, from the point of view of the human sciences, and not the advocacy of particular solutions to particular problems.

5
Individual Aggressiveness and War

IS DESTRUCTIVENESS INBORN?

It is only a short step from consideration of the problems of hostile intergroup feelings, prejudice, and negative discrimination to the question of human conflict and the role of aggressive instinct. The Study Group set out to consider whether current mental health principles could illuminate the present world situation, and took as a starting-point the commonly made statement that destructive aggressiveness is an inborn, instinctual drive in human beings. This traditional viewpoint, manifested in, to take one of many examples, a very common misunderstanding of the now famous UNESCO dictum 'Wars begin in the minds of men', implies, if taken quite literally, that certain combative drives are present in the human psyche that make outbursts of violence and lethal combat inevitable. (In fact, as we understand it, the UNESCO statement implies no such assumption about innate aggressiveness. The minds of men may operate through what is learnt, not necessarily through what is inborn.) The social consequence of such a natural state of inborn combativeness, if it existed, would be that warfare between rival groups was endemic; furthermore, to refer again to the common misunderstanding of the UNESCO phrase, the defences of peace that need to be constructed in the minds of men could be, at best, only temporizing devices. It was cynically remarked of the League of Nations that it was a device to enable the great nations to maintain peace while they thought it suited them.

On the other hand, there is a body of opinion which maintains that there is no such thing as a natural aggressive instinct that leads inevitably to conflict and, through social organization, to war. According to this view, group conflicts occur because of defects in social organization which force human beings into positions from which there is no escape except through fighting.

An anthropologist remarked that it is essential not to confuse the psychodynamics of individuals with the sociodynamics of societies. The existence has been recorded of a number of groups of Homo sapiens among whom war is not known, which suggests the conclusion that war is not an invariable or even an essential aspect of the group adjustment of members of the human species. It might prompt the alternative conclusion that war is a political invention that may even have been forgotten and made afresh many times during human history.

Recent evidence has shown that the great majority of individuals engaged in fighting wars may have little or no aggressive personal motivation of their own. Sample studies made of the UN force during the Korean war revealed that only one in seven of infantry soldiers had actually discharged their weapons under attack. This, the anthropologist pointed out, is a rather dramatic demonstration of a lack of congruence between the fact of belonging to an army and the mobilization of personal aggression.

The initial task for clarification of the discussion is to dissociate theoretically the concepts, first, that mankind is naturally warlike and war is an expression of an ineradicable human instinct; and, second, that man has certain aggressive tendencies responsive to various forms of education, which will be more active under certain social conditions than under others.

Anthropological and sociological evidence heavily supports the position that war is a political invention which, in the past, has served many conflicting interests and has become potentially fatal for the entire human species only since the invention of nuclear and biological weapons. Up to the present day, however much war might be deplored by individuals and however destructive it may have been of particular groups, it has not been lethal to the species.

There is a savage irony in the contemporary dilemma: is it necessary for human beings in general to realize that war can eliminate the human species before warfare can itself be eliminated? And, if so, is it possible to bring about such realization before the species is destroyed?

Discussion of the theoretical questions of whether there is an instinct of destructiveness, as, for example, a death instinct, and what relation such an instinct might have to inherent aggressiveness, appears to be much contaminated by cultural ethnocentrism, signs of which are obvious in theories underlying the practice of child psychiatry, and in parent education and mental health movements in different countries. The various attitudes in different countries cover a wide range, from those that attribute to the child natural evil that has to be brought under control, to those that invest him with natural goodness that is liable to corruption; another view is that the child's mind is a *tabula rasa* on which the individual personality is to be inscribed. Such theories are usually more dependent on historical cultural attitudes towards human nature and on religious sentiment than on objective observation.

These theoretical questions are extremely complex. An anthropologist remarked that to invoke the psycho-analytic theory of instinct relating to destructiveness in order to explain why wars occur may be to confuse a sociocultural problem with one of individual or group psychology. Psycho-analytic theory is more relevant to the motivation of particular individuals who might be in favour of war because they wanted to use it for their own ends, or of certain individuals who enjoy war and may be better adjusted to war than to peace. In endorsing this view, the Study Group emphasized the need to clarify this theoretical position in view of the immense potential of forces of destruction in the modern world.

THE TASK OF RE-EDUCATION

The anthropologist added the idea that today, for the first time in human history in respect of societies of any great size, circumstances have made it imperative that boys be brought up with the conviction that never, in any circumstances, is it permissible to kill another human being. Up to the present time, although every human society has certain taboos or prohibitions in respect of homicide; although boys have everywhere grown up in the conviction that they may not kill their brother, members of their family, or neighbours, or members of the group, tribe, or nation except in certain very restricted and highly specific circumstances, they have everywhere been taught that one day they may be called upon as a duty to kill certain other specified human beings in defence of their own groups. Nowadays the total involvement of the community in war, and the impossibility of restricting the destructiveness of weapons to the permitted categories of victim, have destroyed any value that conventions about destructiveness may once have had.

The immensity of this task of re-education, or, rather, of fundamental redirection of attitude, can be judged by many signs in modern society, for example, the prevalence of violence and homicide as a permitted part of public entertainment on films, television, and so on. The countries of Western Europe and North America (to say nothing of the rest of the world) are very far indeed from the ideal of bringing up boys with the notion that in no circumstances may they ever kill anybody. This crucial question is well within the legitimate field of operational mental health and is one that needs to be urgently considered. Somehow the general realization must be fostered that the methods that have been appropriate to bring up young men who were willing to die for their country must be transformed into methods that will bring up young men who are willing to live and let others live for their country, and to do this in all circumstances and under all forms of provocation. How to do this is known to very few except perhaps the members of certain religious sects or other groups that have existed from time to time.

An educationist pointed to the practical question of devising techniques and methods of minimizing destructive forces both at the level of social organization between groups and at the level of individuals. It is well recognized that in the case of children there is a very close relationship between the manifestation of aggressiveness and the experience they have had of frustration.

One of the educational tasks is to promote more realistic views among the general public of the nature of the angry tendencies and aggressive potential of normal individuals, and recognition of the need to find constructive substitutes for the direct expression of aggressive impulses. In addition, more public recognition is needed of the normality of consciously acknowledging and tolerating the existence of aggressive feelings both in other people and in oneself. This has been well illustrated in those educational circles where it is now recognized that some children may be incapable of learning if no one can accept and tolerate their angry feelings, and that it is not until they meet a teacher who has this capacity of acceptance that they begin to grow and develop. Similarly, many teachers find great difficulty in their work because they have not come to terms with their own anger. The best contribution that mental health can make to these issues is to promote the understanding of the negative valencies that exist in human relations.

ATTITUDES TO MILITARY SERVICE

The experience of military service in various countries throws some light on these issues. An educational psychologist remarked that in Norway, which had not been involved in a major war for 140 years prior to 1940, the period of military service used to be forty days and was not taken seriously. In 1940, at the time of the German invasion, the young men were more than unprepared for warfare, and many were in a state of acute emotional conflict about killing. There were instances of young Norwegian soldiers breaking down in tears when they saw German soldiers being killed by their shooting. But the young soldiers continued to shoot and their behaviour gave an example of emotional conflict between inculcated ideals of not killing and more primitive drives towards self-preservation and the defence of one's country.

Thus the situation may often arise in which the individual fights and kills without necessarily experiencing hostile or even aggressive feelings against his opponent, and, in fact, with strong feelings of remorse about inflicting hurt on fellow human beings. There were many reported instances during World War II of commanders being concerned at the lack of personal aggressiveness or hatred shown by soldiers training for combat. The traditional martial attitude that hatred of the enemy must be inculcated for the sake of military morale persists in the face of innumerable examples during history that a positive attachment to an ideal is a more stable support of morale than hatred of the enemy. During World War II an attempt was made to stimulate hatred in one of the British Army battle-training schools by emphasis on atrocity stories, films of destruction by the enemy and indiscriminate killing of British women and children in air raids, and so on, combined with brutal exhortations and simulated realism in battle-training. Far from raising the morale of the troops in training, this was found to increase the incidence of anxiety breakdown, and the attempt was hurriedly abandoned. Psychiatric opinion at the time was that the breakdowns were caused by a heightening of the conflict between the humanitarian ideals of the troops and their sense of duty, through provocation of aggressive feelings without a corresponding increase of the moral sanction for aggressive action.

There is plenty of evidence that these states of emotional conflict of individuals over aggression have continued after the war. In the case of Norway referred to above, military service has been extended to nineteen months and, perhaps, is taken more seriously there, but there is still a good deal of mental and emotional conflict arising from the opposition of the injunctions 'defend your country' and 'thou shalt not kill'. It has been said that among Norwegian youth there is a very strong tendency to shut out all consideration of such questions as nuclear warfare and to take, instead, an extremely keen interest in the more constructive aspects of the current emergence of new nations in previously colonial areas.

The example of the Norwegian soldiers does not fully illustrate the principle suggested above that boys should be brought up with the conviction that in no circumstances can they ever kill another human being. The possibility was always there for the Norwegian young men that they might have to kill somebody at some time, only it was remote. With this reservation the example is an instructive one.

A psychiatrist thought that the attitude of a country towards military service is not a reliable guide to the quality of the aggressiveness of the people concerned; that compulsory military-training policies may have a closer relationship with the state of the natural defences of the country than with attitudes towards killing. Two neighbouring European countries that have had comparable records throughout history of frequent involvement in national wars – France and Great Britain – have had remarkably different policies about military training. France has had a highly developed system of compulsory military training for a great many years, whereas Great Britain has had compulsory military training only for two periods in its history, both in connexion with a world war, from 1917 to 1919 and from 1938 until the abolition of conscription in 1960.

THE INFLUENCE OF CHILD-REARING PRACTICES

The strategic considerations that may be decisive factors in the case of the great modern nation-state with its agglomeration of peoples and cultures only rarely apply in the case of the community that approximates more closely to a single cultural entity. Among the latter, qualitative differences of individual behaviour and attitudes can be distinguished, as between communities that may be described as warlike, tending to become involved in armed conflict, and those that are more pacific.

It is tempting to trace a connexion between the qualities that are highly prized in a community and its most prevalent child-rearing practices. Thus, martial and warlike peoples generally place a high value on self-control under hardship, pain, and emotional tension, and on the non-acceptance of aggressiveness either in oneself or in other people. The example of Sparta as that of a community dedicated to war is often quoted. The stereotype of the Spartan upbringing is proverbial, signifying the extreme in toughness. It involved the repression of all tenderness and the inculcation of a rigid self-discipline – a strict rejection of aggressiveness, whether in oneself, through self-control in frustration, pain, and rage, or emanating from other people, by instant retaliation.

More pacific peoples, on the other hand, tend to be more accepting of emotional reactions and aggressive impulses in themselves and other people. It should be added that so-called martial people cannot legitimately be credited on this basis alone of originating wars, but rather of possessing certain combinations of qualities that may facilitate a warlike reaction when economic, territorial, or other tensions arise. They may also be more ready than a pacific society to resort to war as an instrument of policy.

As a corrective, an anthropologist argued that the quality of instinctual behaviour most heavily involved in warfare is related less to destructive than to protective aggression; that fear for, rather than of, others, mainly triggers the behaviour. Recent work on animal behaviour supports this contention which, if it were proved to be generally true of human beings, would contribute to the solution of one of the major problems in the world today. Thus, the objective would be not so much that of channelling the destructive aggressive impulses that arise from frustration as of controlling the protective aggressive impulses that arise when country, family, friends, and values are deemed to be threatened. Many examples can be quoted to illustrate the profound difference between destructive and protective aggression, notably that of the behaviour of the Soviet army when fighting in Finland and in Russia, respectively, during the Second World War.

The Study Group considered that much confusion has been caused by a tendency to think about aggression and destruction as if they are practically synonymous, and to regard aggression as being more closely linked with a death instinct than knowledge of the facts justifies. Although it is a commonplace that death instinctual trends may work out both aggressively and destructively, a distinction should be made between these outcomes, though they can serve each other. For example, as a psychiatrist suggested, aggression can be at the service of people who, for quite other reasons, want war. It might be that if it were impossible for aggression to be expressed outwardly on other people, then wars also would not be possible; but it would not follow from this that inborn aggression is a primary factor in causing war.

ATTITUDES TO VIOLENCE

There is much to be learnt in this context from the study of cultures where attitudes to violence differ markedly from those that have been characteristic of Europe over the last 2,000 years. The most often quoted example of a different attitude is that of the Hindu culture with its doctrine of *ahimsa*, or non-violence. This came originally from Buddhist ideals of non-attachment and passivity, but has been institutionalized to a greater degree in Hindu culture than elsewhere. It is a historical fact that the Hindus of India have been among the most pacific of all peoples perhaps for a thousand years, and have come under the domination of successive waves of more warlike peoples. However, even the pacific Hindus have seen their imperialistic and expansionistic days, the most recent of these, historically, being those of the Gupta period, at which time Hinduism was carried militarily throughout Indonesia.

An anthropologist considered the island of Bali to be a particularly interesting example for study. This comparatively small island has had perhaps one of the most pacific cultures in the world. Its religion might be described as a kind of fossilized Hinduism, dating from the end of the first millennium AD, with little change since those days. The people are very pacific, wars and armies unknown, and fighting most uncommon. However, more recently the Balinese have had two periods of savage warfare: the first, in the conquest of the neighbouring island of Lambok; the second, during the Japanese occupation of 1942–45. It has appeared that the effect of hundreds of years of pacifism can be washed out almost overnight when institutions that support the pacific attitude collapse.

This sudden obliteration of the effect of generations of pacifism was shown with even more tragic force at the time of the partition of India and Pakistan, when it has been estimated that some 300,000 people lost their lives in communal fighting. It cannot be doubted that the great mass of the Hindu population of India was, and still is, pacifically minded and that *ahimsa* is highly valued. The immense appeal of the ideal of non-violence was very evident during the long campaign for independence, and it is a military fact that during the first four decades of the twentieth century the British military garrison in India never exceeded 25,000 in a population of the order of three hundred million, and in a country of vast dimensions.

In spite of the pacific nature of the Indian people, it was paradoxically a fact that the establishment of British rule resulted in 150 years of unprecedented peace in the subcontinent, wars having occurred not less frequently in India than in Europe up to the eighteenth century. One explanation of this paradox may be that the Hindu society of India had developed one of the most complicated systems of social role allocation that have been known. This was manifested in the complex ramifications of the caste system. Soldiering had a due place among the various social roles, in the so-called martial classes. Just as had been broadly true of traditional China, Indian society commissioned certain sections to do the fighting on behalf of the whole community, and the vast majority of the population were able to live entirely pacific lives. Thus, when the government organized the martial classes and gave them unity of aim there was no one left to fight in the community, and nothing to fight about.

A very small minority – the Jains – took up a cult attitude in regard to violence and killing. For these people any killing became anathema, a psychological position that is consonant with the repression of strong internal aggressive destructive impulses. In contrast to the cult position, the generally passive attitude of the great mass of caste Hindus is hardly consonant with strong repressive mechanisms to control inherent aggression.

Further confirmation of the view that there were not strong

93

internal control mechanisms can be found in the recruiting experiences in India during the Second World War, when the Indianization of the officer cadre of the Indian army was carried through without difficulty by drawing on the services, freely offered, of young Brahmins, a class of the population not previously regarded as being martial, in fact, quite the reverse. In this case there was more than an external enemy; there was also the prospect of independence to be worked for.

Discussion of these subjects is apt to reveal a certain looseness of use of terms like aggression, hostility, and destructiveness. The term aggression itself, being quite non-commital, merely signifying a movement towards, can be used for any activity that is directed towards an objective. It is presumably because movement towards an instinct-determined objective may, if frustrated, increase in force and become potentially dangerous to obstacles in the way of attainment of instinctual satisfaction that the word aggression has acquired a 'bad' meaning. The more or less incidental destructive effect of the instinctual force that is overcoming an obstacle is often misinterpreted as the actual objective of the movement.

Thus, the individual who is threatened with destruction by an enemy is being faced by the maximum degree of frustration of his instinctual drives towards living. In removing the threat he may kill his enemy, and in this way the aggression that is evoked by the threat to life may itself prove destructive, but as an indirect rather than a direct result.

As a social scientist pointed out, problems are bound to arise from ineffective control of aggression; but the fact that there are people who do not go to war, the fact that some form of compulsory military service has to be introduced in all countries in order to make people go to war even when the safety of the country is threatened, and the fact that it has never been demonstrated that the aggressiveness of individuals and the need to go to war are connected, are all negative evidence relating to the alleged existence of an inherently aggressive drive that will automatically result in war from time to time.

A further point is, as noted above, that it is possible for a community to canalize its fighting into the role of a warrior class, and also, as has been shown in many countries, notably Great Britain, to canalize urges towards combative behaviour into games and sports in which many interpersonal and intergroup hostilities can be expressed.

Naturally, the question of aggressiveness is not limited to combativeness, and the significance of acts of individual violence needs to be considered. Some of these may be explicable in terms of the operation of instinctual mechanisms that are part of social organization. This conclusion is suggested by the findings of studies of herd animals, in which the presence of complex inhibitory mechanisms preventing lethal aggression within the species has been demonstrated. It has been pointed out that neither religious nor cultural influences appear to be decisive in this field, as shown by the savage civil wars of traditional Hindu cultures cited above, and the notorious savagery of religious wars in Europe. In respect of acts of individual aggression within a culture, a psychiatrist reported that a study of hospital admissions in Thailand, a country perhaps more completely expressive of Buddhist teaching than any other, revealed that one-third of the patients in a group of hospitals were occupying beds because they had suffered violence, notably gun-shot wounds or stab wounds. Thailand is a country where aggression is not countenanced, according to religious principles.

THE CONTROL OF AGGRESSIVE TENDENCIES

A biologist called attention to the existence of biological levels at which aggression could be entirely controlled, at least in consciousness, as, for example, the protective concern of parent for child. He added that protective concern of parent for offspring is widely dispersed throughout the animal kingdom, even extending to many classes of insect.

It is broadly true that no animal will kill the young of its own species unless profoundly disturbed, to the extent that any departure from this principle is exceptional. It is also broadly true that adult protectiveness towards the young extends to the young of other species in so far as the young are recognizable as such by the animal. This latter principle is less firmly established than the former, but the fact that it exists at all suggests the presence of powerful influences.

It is characteristic of Homo sapiens that adults feel protective towards all children of whatever nationality, culture, or race. The anthropologist suggested that this virtually universal protective concern of adults for children might be used as a factor in the prevention of war, now that the destructiveness of war has become intolerable for world society. No nation is now able to protect its own young, adequately, from the retaliation of an enemy. Thus any act of warlike aggression will inevitably harm not only the young of the enemy but also (through retaliation) the young of the aggressor. This indisputable fact may be of service in an attempt to harness to the prevention of war the protective concern of adults for children.

But this common denominator of protective concern, or whatever it might be called, it was argued by an anthropologist, cannot be used as a panacea, because it incorporates an oversimplification in not taking account of the capacity of human beings to tolerate the modification, control, and even the frustration of their own instinctual drives. Indeed, such capacity is basic to civilization, but it can take strange and extreme forms, including the capacity of individuals to be extremely cruel to members of their own group. There have been examples of cultures where women, in order to raise their social status, have murdered their babies. At the present time in India, roughly twice as many girl children as boy children die young, but since the same standards of care and nutrition are objectively available to children of both sexes, these differential death-rates can perhaps be regarded as the result of a form of inactive murder of the girls – a form that does not conflict with the doctrine of *ahimsa* to which reference has been made above. Infanticide for various reasons is one of the commonest of the social practices encountered that seem to be directly in opposition to maternal drives. Another aspect of the same phenomenon of withdrawal of empathy and fellow-feeling is the capacity of human beings to regard other human beings as second-class citizens, or even as subhuman, and to embark on the negative discriminatory practices which have been discussed in a previous section.

Observation of animals supports the conclusion drawn from the phenomena discussed above that killings and cruelty within the species are more characteristic of Homo sapiens than of any other species. We must recognize the danger of the potentiality that exists in human beings for the distortion of instinctual processes not only in the direction of the destructive application of aggressiveness, but also in the direction of the defective application of control mechanisms of aggressive impulses. This complex potentiality can have terrible consequences for the individual, his victims, and for the whole of society. Whereas in some societies there has been considerable success in the adaptation of these destructive tendencies to peaceful purposes, in other societies these potentialities have become organized and canalized into destructive ends with very harmful effects, in terms of terrorism and other manifestations of public violence.

History suggests that every society, given the means and the opportunity – including freedom from the compulsion of external aggression – can develop an educational system and a social atmosphere which will result in the control of aggression on the part of almost all of its individual members. But there is no known instance of any human society – not excepting those societies that have no experience of war, those that hunt only for food, and those that are strictly vegetarian – that does not include among its membership some individuals whose aggressiveness has not been successfully controlled. This brings the discussion back to the key point made earlier that, for the prevention of war in the nuclear age, the greatest need is to work towards a universal social ethic which can ensure that no individual will kill another human being in any circumstances whatever.

As the discussion in these pages has shown, the Study Group considered that the presence in the human personality of an inborn or endogenous aggressiveness that makes conflict an inevitable possibility is unproven; but, conceding for the sake of argument the possibility of this hostile element in man's nature, an industrial psychologist urged the importance of distinguishing between reactive and endogenous aggression. The Study Group was impressed by the absence of clear evidence that people normally behave aggressively because of an inner need to do so, regardless of circumstance. There is abundant evidence that it is normal for human beings to act aggressively as a result of the frustration of instinctual drives, and especially in self-defence when threatened. Otherwise, however, it appears to be a universal norm that aggressive behaviour occurs only if certain controls established by socialization have broken down or if such controls have never been set up. An illustration can be taken from some of the African townships in South Africa, where violent behaviour appears to have followed the detribalization process. What appears to have happened there is that the traditional restraints have not been adequately replaced by those current in modern, industrial, urban culture, because African city-dwellers tend to live in a cultural environment which is neither the one nor the other. In these circumstances parents fall back upon instilling fear and physical punishment as the major means of enforcing conformity, with the result that a resort to violence becomes habitual to the developing child.

In the case of this South African example, of course, the issue is not solely one of detribalization: there are other complex factors operating; but there is no lack of other evidence of fluctuations in manifestations of violence. Study of the historical patterns of behaviour in any one country is likely to reveal periods during which violent behaviour has characterized public life, but to various degrees and in different ways at different times and places. Great variations can be found, for example, in the readiness with which violent mobs appear at times of social upheaval. It is likely that every country has had periods in which mob violence has been prevalent – a phenomenon that has currently entirely disappeared from many countries. An excellent historical example can be found in Great Britain where, during the late Middle Ages, at the time of the English baronial wars of the fifteenth century, violence, whether group or individual, was a completely accepted part of so-called civilized life. By the end of the sixteenth century, although national energy and cohesive activity were at a far higher level, violence had become limited and more institutionalized in society. The social acceptability of individual violence had become very restricted; but spontaneous violent group behaviour for political or, at that time, religious ends was still accepted as a social norm which was reflected extensively in drama and literature. During the course of the seventeenth century mob violence largely disappeared from the English scene; it reappeared in attenuated form at very infrequent intervals during the industrial changes of the late eighteenth and early nineteenth centuries.

A postscript may be added to this illustration: since the meeting of the Study Group there have been two widely publicized series of outbreaks of mob violence in Great Britain. The first consisted of a series of incidents in two widely separated localities and spread over a period of one month, in which growing West Indian immigrant local groups were subjected to some personal interference and insult, and suffered damage to property, not so much by local residents as by aggregations of hostile individuals from considerable distances. The strength and rapidity of the public reaction against this outbreak of violence were not the least impressive aspect of the incident.

The second series of incidents occurred in connexion with anti-nuclear-weapon demonstrations, which took an inverted form: the demonstrators adopted the ostensibly non-violent technique of squatting on the ground in public places as a means of forcing their views into public attention. Their passivity effectively neutralized sporadic incidents of mob counter-violence, but the severity of the penalties exacted upon the organizers of the non-violent demonstrators by the legal authorities attracted much criticism at the time. These illustrations show something of changing attitudes to violence in a settled community over a period of several hundred years. Comparable phenomena can probably be found in most cultures.

ANIMAL STUDIES

The current wide range of animal studies in this field does not throw much light on the matter of human group aggression, because the complexity of organization of human society largely invalidates any attempt to apply animal group phenomena to Homo sapiens. Many studies of the behaviour of canine packs have indicated that their territorial conflicts are governed by inhibitory instinctual mechanisms which control aggressive behaviour. In general, the strength of the inhibition has a direct relationship with the distance from the recognized home base, i.e. the further from home the stronger the inhibition. At the risk of oversimplifying, it is tempting to draw here a parallel between this canine behaviour and the well-recognized heightened aggressiveness of human beings when home or cherished values are closely threatened. Apart from territorial defence, in which strong inhibitory mechanisms protect fellow members of the species, in the case of carnivorae the motive for killing is almost exclusively the obtaining of food. Though deaths may occur during struggles for sexual supremacy, these are incidental rather than a direct consequence of fighting. Among herbivorae also, apart from self-defence, killing is generally no more than incidental to mating struggles, in which the objective is to gain the mate and to drive away rather than destroy a rival. It might be argued that to kill in circumstances other than the above is a pathological act, even among the most savage animals.

A psychiatrist member of the Group recalled observing a territorial fight between two family groups of monkeys in which, apparently, there was some evidence of tactical cooperation between the members of the same family, but the objective of this struggle was to establish a right to the territory rather than to kill members of the other group.

The pacific nature of that much-studied animal, the dolphin, has been recognized for many centuries. There are comments in the writings of Aristotle[1] and of Pliny[2] about the gentle and kindly dolphin, which apparently never acts aggressively towards other animals, except in food-seeking behaviour and occasional action in self-defence, when it has been recorded that a dolphin can kill a shark that is bigger than itself. It has also been recorded lately that in the course of 'training', dolphins do not react aggressively even to the quite brutal treatment that has been described.

THE CHILD AND AGGRESSIVENESS

In the absence of reliable evidence to the contrary, the Study Group thought it might be generally agreed that the problem of war does not lie primarily in individual psychology, but in group and cultural factors. Even so, it may be conceded that the question of aggression in individuals has an essential bearing on the corresponding group phenomena. A child psychiatrist pointed out that the question of aggression cannot be judged without reference to the processes by which the young child gains control of his outward-turning aggressive impulses, to the modification of the instinctual drives that this implies, and to the quality of the reception by his parents of such aggressiveness as he may show.

Child psychiatrists are very familiar with problems caused not only by the uncontrolled aggression of children and the relationship difficulties that follow, but also by the apparent lack of aggression of some children, whether this be by reason of absence of aggression, or of inhibition and over-control. Out of clinical experience one might advance a concept of healthy aggressiveness. Eighteenth-century surgeons used to talk about 'laudable pus' – in the septic conditions of the time, evidence of the body's capacity to react to minor infection by pus formation in wounds was, rightly, taken as a good omen for healing. By analogy we would advance a concept of 'laudable aggressiveness', the re action to minor frustration being a good augury of the strength and organization of normal aggressive drives.

[1] Aristotle, *Hist. Animalium*, IX, 48.   [2] Pliny, *Hist. Nat.*, IX, 8.

A child psychiatrist quoted a case of a child of three who had been brought up in an atmosphere from which all aggressive manifestations had been deliberately and conscientiously excluded, and whose behaviour at home had been quite untroubled. On mixing for the first time in a nursery group, the child received a slap from an aggressive neighbour and was clearly puzzled by this; a second slap resulted in the child dissolving into tears. He appeared to be unable to cope with other children and developed a stutter. It was considered that these developments could be related directly to the child's first experience of aggressive behaviour, and they had to be dealt with by therapy.

It will no doubt be generally agreed that the question of control and direction of aggression is complex and covers a wide range of phenomena: on the one hand is the child who is apparently without aggressive drives because he has never experienced the aggression of others, or has no knowledge of frustration; on the other is the child who has developed inhibitory mechanisms. This type of reaction may have been brought about by the excessive control of the parents, which has caused the child to contain its outward-turning aggressive impulses to the extent that the latter are elicited only when an excessively high level of stress or frustration is experienced. Then the resulting outburst of aggression may be extremely frightening to the child both because of its unfamiliarity – since the child literally has no experience of or practice in controlling his feelings – and because of its excessive force. A vicious circle may be established of over-control and increase of tensions, which causes a compulsive aggressiveness that itself raises the anxiety level and increases the pressure to control. However, such compulsive aggression, being an intensely individual phenomenon, can hardly be regarded as responsible for organized conflict between groups.

THE ELIMINATION OF WAR

The Study Group was agreed that the balance of evidence justified the view that the problem of the elimination of war is not so much that of changing essential human nature as that of modifying those controls of normal human drives that are subject to cultural influences. Although it is a biological truism that infants today begin life with much the same equipment with which infants have been beginning life for 10,000 years – the evidence of genetic mutations in psychological traits being unclear, to say the least – and although in this sense one must agree with the many people who say that 'you cannot change human nature', this is not at all the same thing as saying 'you cannot change the patterns of human behaviour'.

An anthropologist remarked that this is a matter not so much of trying to make people more peaceful or more intelligent as of attempting to build a culture in which it is possible for human beings to learn to behave more peacefully or more intelligently or more responsibly, or to become more generous, or to include more people within their own definition of humanity. In this connexion the notion of greater emotional maturity is often employed, but the Study Group was concerned to promote a new concept of human social and psychological evolution that is free from the notion of maturity as normally used in the study of the development of young animals.

Much of the conceptual difficulty in this area appears to be caused by undisciplined analogical thinking. Thus, uncontrolled violence is frequently linked with the concept of emotional immaturity – for example, the anticipated temper tantrums of the frustrated toddler child. It follows that there is a tendency to define emotional maturity according to the accepted standards of adult behaviour in the particular culture of the individual, with the result that behaviour which is thought of as being inferior to accepted standards is regarded as less emotionally mature. The use of the concept of maturity implies the existence of a normal pattern of human emotional development which is hardly established in respect of individual development in the case of any single culture, and which certainly has no relevance and no established meaning in terms of group behaviour phenomena.

In the example given above of the changing attitude to public violence over the last five hundred years in Great Britain, it is quite erroneous (though it is frequently done by implication) to regard the anarchy of the Middle Ages as analogous to early childhood and seventeenth-century ebullience as a kind of cultural adolescence. This is obviously meaningless, yet the use of the concept of emotional maturity in the assessment of social relationships entails precisely this kind of thinking. It is scientifically more valid to regard the attitude towards violence or social irresponsibility that characterized sixteenth-century Great Britain as simply different from that which characterized the eighteenth century or is current today. If human aggressiveness is conceived of as corresponding to an inherent pattern of human development, any attempt to devise educational means to evolve attitudes that are thought to be desirable will be logically inhibited from the start. This is an example of false analogical thinking that has done great harm. If we adopt more realistic attitudes, the attempt to eradicate war can be kept free from the inevitable pessimism of those who believe that in order to succeed they have to run counter to an aspect of man's essential nature. Instead we can gain benefit from the optimism of those who are aware of man's capacity for adaptation.

6

Fear of Nuclear Destruction

In a working paper, Aase Skard referred to the state of fear
that exists at the present time in all countries open to the instruments of mass communication – the press, radio, television.
There are, almost daily, items of information about nuclear explosions and tests, and acts of aggression by one community
against another.[1] She pointed out that the anxiety aroused by
such information is not necessarily expressed in open symptoms
but can be indirectly expressed or, in some cases, suppressed.

'One may find a general and exaggerated interest in *material*
things (higher material standard of life by gadgets, by cars,
refrigerators, etc.) and in social competition as expressed in
material matters (the newest car, the most expensive mix-
master), and/or diminishing interest in political and social
questions with increasing feeling of irresponsibility in national
and international problems. Or one may find an attitude of
"eat, drink and be merry for tomorrow we die" with increase of alcoholism, lack of sexual control, and decreasing
sympathy with others. On the other hand, the fear of a possible catastrophe may add itself to already existing anxieties in
the individual, and drive him towards suicide, mental breakdown, or other forms of imbalance. (It goes without saying
that unconscious anxieties may also be projected on the actual
source of fear.)'

[1] Since the date of this working paper (1961) the number of news
items concerning weapon-testing has decreased as a result of an international agreement about tests. However, the threat of disaster,
as reflected in the mass media, remains scarcely less imminent for
all of those countries involved in nuclear activity, and for their neighbours.

She posed three questions:

(i) How far should people be encouraged to experience and express their fear consciously?

(ii) To what extent can 'fear of the fear' be alleviated without provoking a pathological degree of anxiety?

(iii) How can people be helped to deal with their fears about the present world situation in constructive ways, without invoking one of the harmful mechanisms to which she referred above?

The Study Group's discussion in this area was primarily concerned with the competence of mental health workers to handle the all-important current (1961) anxiety about the immense potential destructiveness of the hydrogen bomb.

THE RISK CAUSED BY PSYCHOPATHOLOGY

As a starting-point, the Group considered some of the possibilities of disaster being precipitated by the presence of psychopathological conditions among those who are dealing with nuclear weapons. In a working paper, Fox pointed out that it might be possible for a mentally ill person to induce healthy colleagues to act upon his delusions; that social isolation and conditions of stress are particularly conducive to shared delusions of the kind that have been excellently described in the novel *The Caine Mutiny*. The conditions under which people handling nuclear weapons are working appear commonly to engender stress from isolation. Psychiatrists recognize that paranoid states tend to be insidious in origin and that, without anyone else being aware of the fact, a paranoid person may long incubate plans for retribution against imaginary persecutors, or against influences conceived to be malign, or may nurse designs to save himself, his family, his country, or mankind.

Another psychological disorder that can be dangerous in this setting is one that occurs occasionally in cases of severe depression, in which the individual projects his depressive feelings upon those with whom he has an emotional relationship. There is a great deal of experience in psychiatric practice of the depressed patient who kills other people in the course of a dramatic suicide, or who commits murder as an act of supposed mercy. It is not being unreasonably imaginative to point to the possible danger of such pathological psychological dynamisms operating among lonely and exposed people who are bearing the burden of responsibility for operating nuclear-weapon systems. The question of how to make a missile-release system proof against individual psychopathology is, the Study Group contended, very much within the field of mental health interest; of equal concern are the possible effects of the secrecy that surrounds such arrangements. It is obvious that no chain of command can be completely immune to human fallibility.

The communication of delusional systems, whether through *folie à deux* or through the working-out of other disordered rationalizations, is a highly dangerous possibility in this field. Another serious factor is that many people who are without apparent mental illness have arrived at the belief, to which we have referred above, that nuclear war is inevitable sooner or later. They may have been influenced by historical arguments, which may themselves be no more than rationalizations of an underlying state of anxiety; but once this conclusion has been reached, the reaction may be the thought that the sooner one gets going the better the chance of victory.

To the risks of disaster arising from individual or shared mental illness or anxiety-distorted judgement must be added the accidents that may occur through misinterpretations of evidence and false alarms. Again, the anxiety prevalent in the population because of knowledge that such accidents are possible is a mental health consideration. It does not require competence in one of the mental health disciplines to lead one to the conclusion that, in this area, the danger of panic action occurring is severe. Even in the past, with greatly inferior means of mass communication, a prophecy of the end of the world, made by some self-appointed prophet or based on a calculation from the dimensions of the pyramids of Egypt, or the predictions of a Nostradamus, have been sufficient to send whole groups of people to the desert or to the tops of mountains to await the moment of doom. How much greater is the danger of widespread panic today!

THE PROTEAN QUALITY OF NUCLEAR ANXIETY

It is clear that conditions of danger tend to be self-sustaining, in that human reactions to danger tend to intensify the dangerous state. An anthropologist illustrated this point by reference to happenings in California in 1961, when groups of teenagers had been stealing explosives and storing them away in the hills against an anticipated seizure of power by communists. It is to be presumed that if tension in this area were to become sufficiently great other groups would begin to store explosives against the anti-communists. Indeed, this is the traditional situation of the arms race which, in the opinion of historians, has in the past always led to warfare. Wherever there is social tension, and wherever people begin to arm themselves against a possible eventuality, the likelihood of the disastrous eventuality's occurring is greatly increased. Anxiety on this score is very much in people's minds as they witness the competition between the powers equipping themselves with nuclear weapons.

We do not know enough about what ordinary people in various countries are thinking and fantasying about nuclear weapons and all that they signify. Although it is commonly stated that there is a great deal of public anxiety about such matters as nuclear-testing and radio-active fall-out, the evidence (such as it is) appears to be more impressive to the contrary – i.e. it suggests that the greater tendency is for people not to think about these problems. In other words, it appears likely that the familiar mental mechanisms of repression, displacement, rationalization, and over-compensation are occurring to a considerable extent. A psychiatrist remarked that when, in the course of analytic treatment, the atom bomb appeared in a patient's dreams, it tended to appear as a symbol of a personal situation and seemed to have little direct connexion with the world situation. The Study Group considered that this is an area of mental health in which far more work should be done; it is one in which very little scientific work has been published.

In 1957 the World Health Organization set up a study group on 'Mental Health Aspects of the Peaceful Uses of Atomic Energy' (532). This interdisciplinary group considered some of the anxiety-creating aspects of the subject. The mandate of the group was strictly limited to considering the peaceful uses of atomic energy, but it was immediately apparent that anxiety focused on nuclear weapons could not be sharply distinguished from the general state of anxiety relating to the whole field of atomic research. Although a number of years have elapsed without the feared disaster occurring, and although slow and partial progress has been made towards international agreement, the anxiety of ordinary people, though less consciously articulate, perhaps, appears to be generally as strong as ever and prone to be triggered off by quite minor events. We believe that the WHO report is still very topical.

The WHO study group noted that, as far as information was available, everything connected with the subject of atoms provokes a strong reaction which, however, varies greatly according to the different levels or social groups in a society. But whereas nuclear explosions almost everywhere command banner headlines in newspapers, the subject is just as apt to empty as to fill a hall if public discussion is attempted – a reaction that may be due to the apathy which many people experience when they feel that a situation is beyond their control and that nothing can be done about it.

The published report (1958) noted how much atomic matters have entered into people's day-to-day conversation. There was a phase when everything disagreeable was freely blamed on the atom bomb – bad weather, natural disasters, the failure of a harvest. This kind of reaction may be less manifest now, owing to habituation, but there is still a good deal of expressed anxiety about fall-out or the disposal of atomic waste, and the pollution of water and milk supplies. There are also unresolved fears of sterility and of harmful genetic effects.

One of the most striking reactions to be found is that of confusion of thought. Many people appear to pass from confusion
and mistrust to a condition of apathy that makes them incapable
of thinking about the subject. As the Director of the Medical
Division of Atomic Energy of Canada Limited has remarked:
'A good many people consider anything connected with atomic
energy to be something that can well be, and probably is, extremely dangerous. . . . A large segment of the public appears
to be fully convinced that it would be quite unable to understand
the simple fundamental principles of atomic energy.'

In a survey conducted by the American Institute of Public
Information in February 1956, about half the sample interviewed
were unable to say anything in answer to the question, 'Do you
know of any uses for atomic energy other than for war purposes?'

An inquiry made by the WHO study group concerning the
appearance of nuclear fantasies in psychotic symptomatology
gave, it was stated, a 'surprisingly blank result'. It was recognized that in the history of psychiatry the symptoms of psychosis
have included a series of 'influences' – ranging from hypnotism,
through various forms of mechanical power, to electricity, radio,
and so on – incorporated into the patients' delusional systems,
usually with a strong fear content. Whereas radar had been freely
incorporated into delusional systems, nuclear energy had entered
only very rarely, and since the notion of nuclear energy is older
than that of radar, this finding deserves increased research
attention.

The WHO study group remarked upon the extraordinarily protean character of the anxieties that can be aroused by the idea of
nuclear weapons. This has been reflected in science fiction which,
during the present century, has steadily stressed the horrors of
scientific power. A notable example was the 'death ray', a classical
fantasy of horror fiction a generation ago, which, it may be noted,
is still an object of scientific activity. More recently there has
been a widespread superman-type of fantasy in so-called comics
and other publications for the semi-literate: a human being
assumes magical powers in order to defeat the horrors of science.

In many parts of the modern world, with the shrinking of communications and the current fantasy of the penetrative powers of destructive influences, it is keenly felt that there is no safe place and nowhere to hide.

The WHO study group discussed some of the peculiar qualities of nuclear energy from which the more protean fantasies are derived. It was reflected that radiation is 'invisible, unheard, unsmelt, untasted, and unfelt, apparently infinitely powerful, yet springing from an almost infinitely small source, and – as far as the individual is concerned – uncontrollable'.

'Of all these aspects the most terrifying and most characteristic is perhaps that of a tremendous power that may get out of control. . . . In the 1920s – the heyday of the death-ray period of science fiction . . . there was a widespread terrifying fantasy of the splitting of the atom which would set off the unstoppable nuclear chain reaction that would go on splitting atoms and so compass the destruction of the universe.

In the 1950s, when the fear of the physical chain reaction has been proved groundless, the non-scientific public has fostered another fear, the fear of the biological chain reaction. It is, for example, expressed as a fear that fall-out or atomic waste may damage algae, which in turn will damage waterplants, and then fish, and eventually humans – above all, their genes. This is a deeper and more subtle fear than that of the unleashing of energy that might destroy the universe. . . .'

The WHO study group drew an analogy between the situation of man in relation to atomic power and the situation of the very young child first experiencing the world – an analogy that the group recommended for serious technical study. One of the most protean of the anxieties invoked is that of man's anxiety about his own search for knowledge and for power, an anxiety that is reflected almost universally in myth and legend. For example, Prometheus unlawfully not only came to understand fire, but appropriated it, the prerogative of the gods, for the use of man, and suffered terrible punishment; Pandora also brought disaster to the world by tampering with the prerogative of the gods; and Faust incurred disaster through assuming the powers of God. The association of knowledge with evil and punishment is explicitly set out in the story of the Garden of Eden, and also in an ancient Egyptian saying, quoted by the WHO study group: 'When man learns what moves the stars, the sphinx will laugh and life will be destroyed.'

In development of this analogy it was pointed out that every child is born helpless, and dependent upon powers that are, relative to him, apparently infinite; all-providing but unpredictable; the source of almost infinite benefits or the possible cause of ultimate destruction. Clinical evidence suggests that children who are in conflict with parental power are prone to destructive fantasies (including that of self-destruction).

Another source of anxiety in young children is how to control their own capacity for aggressive action. Aggression is used here in the neutral sense referred to above – as one of the great universal forces of mankind, without which survival would be inconceivable. The individual child must gain control of his natural aggressiveness if he is not going to be destroyed by it or by the effect of his uncontrolled aggression upon his environment. The gaining of a high degree of control promotes the child's confidence and feeling of security, but forces that appear uncontrollable are a potent cause of anxiety to the individual.

Clinical evidence in the case of children shows that, where there is not perfect security, the infant's situation of weakness in the face of powers that, relative to him, may appear to be omnipotent is apt to arouse the most intense anxiety of a very primitive character. In the face of the threat of the atomic bomb, the individual man is placed like the infant in a situation of maximum weakness at the mercy of impersonal or, what is worse, apparently malign, omnipotence. Just as the over-anxious child universally shows regression to infantile behaviour and modes of thinking, so the ordinary man, confronted with the terrifying image of nuclear destruction, demonstrates all manner of irrational thought and behaviour.

EVIDENCE OF REGRESSION IN PUBLIC REACTIONS

Evidence of regressed attitudes is almost universal, as shown by the anxiety expressed in press coverage of atomic items. A scrutiny of the world's press made by the WHO study group revealed an intense excitability about the whole subject. A more concrete example of regressed attitudes, both in the ordinary man and woman and in the authorities, can be seen in the various civil disobedience campaigns that have been conducted in a number of countries in connexion with nuclear weapons.

In quoting this example, it is emphasized that there are many countries in which popular demonstrations are suppressed, and that the first essential for the existence of a civil disobedience campaign is a constitution in which public expressions of dissidence against governmental policy are possible, for which an atmosphere of political sophistication is essential. In such an atmosphere, examples of regressed attitudes and behaviour are all the more striking.

For example, in 1961 in the United Kingdom, there were a number of public demonstrations against nuclear weapons which took the form of 'squatting' in public places, with the avowed object of drawing dramatic public attention to the aims of the organizers of the protest, and to that extent embarrassing the government of the day. On one particular Saturday afternoon, a crowd, variously estimated at several thousand, by prearrangement sat down in the road in Whitehall, the London street that symbolizes government and leads to the Houses of Parliament. The time being Saturday afternoon, and the district being well served with connecting streets, it might well be asked who was being inconvenienced by this gesture, which symbolized infantile dependence in no uncertain terms.

The authorities had been given warning of the intention of the demonstrators; they mobilized several thousand policemen and several hundred vehicles, and literally carried more than 1,500 demonstrators to vehicles, from whence they were taken into hastily improvised magistrates' courts and charged with obstructing the highway. Small fines were inflicted and paid by all except a small minority of more intrepid demonstrators who elected to take the alternative short period of imprisonment. From the point of view of a student of human behaviour, it appears to be a moot point which party was behaving in the more regressed way – the self-appointed infants who squatted in the street, or the authorities who ordered the 'nurses' to carry away the infants and administer the dose.

THE CHANGING BALANCE OF POLITICAL POWER

The WHO study group drew attention to a further source of new and increased anxieties which has accompanied the introduction of nuclear weapons, namely that the balance of power between political leaders, military leaders, and scientists has been changed beyond restitution. Few political leaders in any country have a background of scientific training, yet they are called upon to make decisions in situations which, to an increasing degree, have been built up by the work of scientists, and which, for proper handling, more and more require some conception of the implications of scientific work. Lack of an adequate conceptual background can lead to a crippling insecurity, which generates uncertainty about who actually wields the power, and how; and anxiety about the moral implications of research into weapons heightens the tension.

Traditionally, the seat of executive power in the state has been with political leaders, who have had control of the instruments of power – the armed forces. This arrangement has, on the whole, been effective because of a general understanding by the politicians of the potentialities and limitations of the power wielded by the military leaders. This political control extended also in general terms to weapon research; furthermore, those undertaking research into the more lethal types of weapon have, at least up to the end of the nineteenth century, been the same people as those who have had responsibility for using the weapons in the field, and have been personally among those exposed to retaliation from the enemy.

The introduction of nuclear weapons has transferred the control of these weapons – which entirely overshadow all other armaments – absolutely into the hands of a very small group in each country, composed of those scientists who, alone in the community, understand both how to manufacture the weapons and how to use them. The dependence of both politicians and military leaders on the scientist is now absolute in respect of nuclear weapons and, what is more, the political leaders are also entirely dependent on their scientific advisers in estimating the strengths and dangers of the situation of their own country, and the potentialities of enemies. In spite of these radical changes there has been little or no change in the chain of responsibility and power during the present century.

The dependence of political leaders on others in the community, especially upon the military, is not new. From ancient times countries have devised formal or social institutions to control powerful people in the community. The standard pattern of social institution has entailed a strong emphasis on discipline, obedience, and loyalty, and a hierarchy of authority within both the civil and the military services, so that all are subordinated to the ultimate seat of authority in the state. This discipline and obedience constitute a total attitude of mind that is inculcated in professional civil servants and military personnel; it is not introduced from their first moment of service, rather, it is in the family traditions of the social groups from which they are drawn. Thus, the political leader is in a position to count with certainty on the loyalty and obedience of those with whom he is to work, and who exercise the power in the state on his behalf.

In the nuclear age, however, the members of this political-civil-military hierarchy are themselves dependent upon the technologist, who has no tradition of service and may have no inculcated pattern of loyalty to the ruling system. The scientist who has been brought up in an abstract discipline of science may have as his primary basic value the duty to follow scientific processes regardless of the moral consequences.

Thus, the pure or abstract scientist who continues to give himself to a scientific pursuit, though well aware that his work will be used ultimately for the preparation of weapons of destruction, represents a new phenomenon in the history of the human community. Whereas at one time the man who devised the weapons was among those likely to be killed by them, the scientist today, because of his estimated value to the community in time of war, is the most likely to be protected. When his aim is the perfection of a technological device, irrespective of the moral consequences of his work, his social role can be regarded as, at best, irresponsible and, at worst, criminal.

THE PREDICAMENT OF THE ORDINARY INDIVIDUAL

These are complex psychological and moral issues which require far more exhaustive treatment than is possible in the present discussion. Our aim here is to do no more than draw attention to some of the probable consequences of these modern developments. The various countries engaged in atomic warfare research are no doubt trying to solve these political and social dilemmas in their characteristic ways. What is common to the whole world is that ordinary men and women are kept in a state that is worse than ignorance because of the primitive fantasies and wild rumours to which they are continuously subjected. The situation is made worse by the much publicized secrecy that surrounds installations, and the various rumours and speculations as to how 'the other side' manages these things. It is said, for example, that the atomic experts are held in a state of dependence on the political authority in that no single individual has the key to the whole process, and that it is within the power of only one person, designated by the political power, to complete the chain of events by which the nuclear weapon can be activated. This is only one example of the kind of speculation that is rife, and it reveals the prolific character of the fantasy that permeates this field.

Reviewing these matters, the WFMH Study Group considered it not surprising that such uncertainties and anxieties about survival are reflected in human behaviour. Among the various reports brought by members of the Group, it was said that in the United States, for example, the younger people showed a greater tendency to 'eat, drink and be merry, for tomorrow we die' while there was an impression that the older people in the community observed a considerable degree of silence on these topics. Similar tendencies were reported in Scandinavia where, on the whole, people appear to try not to think of these matters, or to treat them as something very far off, and a minority show a strong desire to enjoy life while they still have it. Others unconsciously limit their lives to narrow horizons and keep within their own social setting, and, for example, may become very preoccupied with the building of a new house.

Anxiety over survival, on a world-wide basis, has been a characteristic and growing phenomenon of the present century. The generation that had reached maturity at the outbreak of the Second World War spent its early childhood during the First World War, had been profoundly shocked by the unprecedented mortality and savagery of that war, and had tried passionately to believe that this had been 'the war to end war'. Fear of the recurrence of world conflict and horror of the increasing strength of weapons had been constant anxieties of a whole generation. At the outbreak of World War II in 1939, vast numbers of people in Europe had been led to believe from military pronouncements that the power of high explosive was so great that big cities could be annihilated in a single raid. Repeated experience of bombing in 1940 and 1941 convinced people that this was not true, but gave them nevertheless a terrifying experience of the possibilities of explosives, and strengthened the feeling that if it were not true today it might well be true in a few years' time; in any case, the feeling was confirmed by the nuclear bombing of Hiroshima and Nagasaki. It is not much comfort to people faced with a critical situation to learn that, historically, such fears have always been expressed, and that, no doubt, the inventors of gunpowder in their day, as far as the limited communications allowed, suffered execration like the inventors of nuclear weapons in the twentieth century.

Whatever the individual reaction to the anxiety situation, it is clear that the whole thinking and feeling tone of the current generation has been coloured by the prospect of possibilities of cosmic disaster. An anthropologist remarked that the mental health angle on this problem goes much further than merely an attempt, by putting oneself in the position of belonging to another country or party, to understand the situation from someone else's viewpoint, useful though this is in its own right. We have a responsibility also to put ourselves in the position of other generations. The Study Group, thinking of the enormous changes taking place in the patterns of life, considered that it is imperative that those engaged in mental health work should put themselves in the position of the twenty-year-olds and attempt to work out how the current world appears to them. This attempt needs to be made afresh, on the spot, and not just as a matter of speculation based on memories of what things felt like during the youth of the middle-aged observer.

There is a great need to make comparative studies between countries as to what the younger generation thinks and feels about the nuclear age. For example, it would be instructive to compare French youth today, growing up in a country that has been closely involved in an almost continuous experience of warfare for centuries, with the youth of other countries that have been more remote from war, or with those of countries that have been in close proximity to but not actually engaged in warfare, like Sweden and Switzerland. It was reported that in the United States there has lately been among the middle classes a spread of a form of behaviour that is traditionally associated with the insecure and poor of the community – i.e. living for the day, buying on the instalment plan, and neither planning nor saving for the future. This type of behaviour is customarily thought of as lower-class behaviour and its spread is sometimes attributed to the rise of the concept of the welfare state; but perhaps it could be attributed with greater accuracy to widespread insecurity about the future.

THE RATIONAL FEAR OF TOTAL DISASTER
The Study Group agreed with the view expressed by an anthropologist that it would be a very serious source of error to suppose

that the anxiety about destruction during World War I or World War II could be fairly compared with the present anxiety. The present situation is fundamentally different in that never before within the consciousness of the people has there been a rational fear of a total holocaust. In the past, certain groups have been wiped out where they failed to take or initiate particular actions, but as far as anthropological or historical evidence can take us, no group of human beings in the past has been consciously aware of the possibility of total destruction about which they can do nothing. This is the first time in history that man has known that he possesses the power of total destruction, though, of course, it is not the first time that there have been prophets of impending doom. Such prophecies have been made throughout history – probably whenever novel types of war machine have been invented, or new techniques of destruction – but up to the present time the ascertainable facts have never justified the terms of the prophecy. This time the facts do appear to fit the prophecy.

The anthropologist reported that some young people feel frustrated because their seniors do nothing except talk about banning the bomb. These young people feel that a ban could not solve the problem, because, as far as they can tell, whatever they may feel or do, they are condemned to live, if not with the stockpile, which could be destroyed, then with the knowledge that the bomb could be made by many people at any time. It may be contended that this view is neither pessimistic nor apathetic, but realistic; that these young people have understood the essential difference between the present situation and the historical one.

After considerable discussion, the Study Group agreed that the strong emphasis placed upon the elements of change in the current situation is justified. Man's preoccupation with fantasies of destruction, which has been particularly marked at the conclusion of each major war, has led people to think each time that the world has been essentially changed, that a new generation has been born during the war, and the destructiveness of the next war has been fantasied in exaggerated terms. But always, hitherto, there has been a conviction that the facts do not fit the most gloomy prognostications. There has also been a belief – which may not be at all objective – that defence measures are not far behind weapons of offence; that for every evil there is a remedy. Now it appears there are no such convictions and beliefs among those who are facing the situation squarely, and it is their view that the problem that now faces humanity is how to live with imminent potential destruction.

A psychologist referred to another change which, though not so fundamental as the above, is nonetheless significant. The impact of the revolutions which followed World War I during the interwar period gave many young people in countries all over the world a feeling of being part of a process of change which was, nevertheless, manageable, because the world retained, in outward structure at least, familiar forms and familiar balances of relationship. The great ferment of social change set in train by the disturbances of World War II has had a more fundamental quality. The nuclear bomb has upset the balance of power in the world, and created new power structures. Dramatic changes in world-leadership patterns have been created by the newly emerging states. These newer states are troubled by uncertain and conflicting goals; the older states are thinking in terms of retreat and unmanageable change. Those accustomed in the past to be leaders in the cultural and other spheres are uncertain about their role in the future, and unclear about the new images that are being created. Among such people a predominant feeling is one of helplessness. What can one do? What goals can one have?

Once again such phenomena are not new in the history of civilization. These kinds of feeling must have accompanied every major change that has taken place in political and cultural forms, but there is an essential difference, as in the case of the anxiety in respect of nuclear weapons, in the widespread awareness of the nature of change and of the possibility that life may take on different forms. At the overthrow of the Roman Empire or at the fall of Constantinople, it is to be supposed that only a very small group of those who were philosophically and historically minded can have had any insight into what was happening. The great mass of the defeated people would feel simply that all that they valued in life had been overwhelmed. At the present time, with a great spread of insight and knowledge concerning other ways of life and other cultures, the problem affecting a much higher proportion of the population is how to learn to live with the unfamiliar present and an uncertain future.

CONCLUSIONS

The Study Group concluded its discussion of this subject by reaching agreement on a statement which had been prepared by one of its members for inclusion in the summary report of this International Study Group, *Mental Health in International Perspective* (21):

'While it is hard to see how psychiatrists can yet give much help in political decisions on the use, abandonment, or control, of weapons of annihilation, they have the duty of warning the world how readily a major disaster may occur even without the intention of any government. In particular, it is important to point out the possible role, in this connexion, of shared psychopathology, more often described clinically as *folie à deux*. Onc mentally disordered person suffering from a delusional state may induce his more stable colleagues to accept his delusions, and to act upon them.

Social isolation and conditions of stress are particularly conducive to shared delusions, and such situations are obviously inherent in nuclear-powered submarines, remote rocket sites and listening posts, and long-range bombing planes.

The psychiatric patient who develops a paranoid delusional state may appear to be of previously normal personality, and the onset of the disorder may be insidious, and undetectable even by his family and friends. While such people are rarely of any danger, their delusions are sometimes of a messianic nature, the patient possibly believing that he will be the saviour of mankind if, for example, he can but ensure the launching of a missile. Or he may wish to achieve this as retribution for imaginary persecution by "spies", "radioactivity", or other malign influences. A variety of similar disordered rationalizations are readily conceivable – and it may be noted that some people, even without apparent mental disorder, believe that a nuclear war is inevitable, and that the sooner one "gets going", the better the chance of victory.

It is a solemn thought that a person in one of these categories might be in a position of responsibility, for, however foolproof a missile-release system may be, if it is to function swiftly it is very hard to imagine that it would be immune to the deliberate plans of an intelligent and determined paranoid individual in a key position, still less to a group of men with a collective psychosis. Again, it is obviously not publicly known how foolproof, in fact, these arrangements are: there may well be far more foundation for these fears than we have been allowed to know.

To the risk of accidental explosion due to individual or shared mental illness must be added accidental hazard – again a subject of which the public is ignorant, although it has been reliably reported that, already on several occasions, "false alarms" have led to the actual mobilization of nuclear weapons. Clearly, the release of missiles depends on a chain of mechanical functions and human assessments, all of which must necessarily be subject to inherent error, breakdown, or misinterpretation. As more countries develop lethal techniques, the risk involved becomes multiplied many times.

This group has, I think, the competence to emphasize these matters frankly and without ideological bias, in the hope that all governments may be stimulated to reach agreement, with greater urgency, on the control of armaments; for, as long as these instruments of destruction exist, every single life hangs by a thread at every moment of every day.'

To this lucid statement it need only be added that those who are working in the mental health field are committed to the high value of sharing and pooling the skills they possess in the field of the human sciences, for human welfare in the widest possible sense. The temptation to make general pronouncements about mental health principles of action should, however, be firmly avoided, and each situation as it arises should be approached on its own merits. Our preoccupation at all times should be to see what positive contribution can be made from our areas of competence.

PART TWO

Problems of Conceptualization

7

Conceptualization of Mental Health

The Study Group early became aware both of a feeling of pressure to arrive at a clear definition of what is meant by the term 'mental health', and of the extreme difficulty of achieving any such formulation. Although it may be conceded that many of the arguments employed against making any attempt to define mental health are derived mainly from the realization of the inadequacy of our background knowledge, at the same time it may be argued that some of the pressure for making a definition is itself the result of unclear thinking.

Some of the major difficulties in the field of biology have been caused by the employment in that field of methods, concepts, and semantics that originated in philosophy and have been developed for use in the physical sciences. Thus, though it is legitimate, and necessary for the sake of communication, to seek clarity and definition in the use of philosophical terms in both abstract and concrete contexts, yet in the field of living matter, such definitions, where they can be applied, are necessarily less precise than in the field of organic science. It is a logical impossibility to make any finite definition of a living organism whose future history is still unknown. Where dynamic, abstract concepts are included in the field of study the pressure to arrive at definitions is even less relevant.

At the meeting of the International Preparatory Commission in 1948, a psychologist member threw the discussion into confusion by posing the question: 'What do you mean by mental health?' However, the Commission accepted this question as legitimate; and since that time mental health literature has manifested a certain defensiveness about a growing consciousness of the inability to define the term 'mental health'. This defensiveness, it may be thought, results from recognition of the clear need of those who interpret mental health concepts to a wider public to be able to use terms that are properly understood.

In our view, suggested definitions of mental health have hitherto proved unsatisfactory because they were attempting an impossible task, and we would question whether, in the field of human behaviour, it is reasonable to try to proceed at an early stage to the formulation of definitions. The point may be further illustrated by an analogy taken from biology. The definition of an elephant, in the strict tradition of the philosophical and natural sciences, relates to the natural order, genus, and species. Any additional information about the animal goes beyond a definition into the field of an operational description. The definition by itself does not enable the individual to recognize the phenomenon unless he has a profound knowledge of the subject and can use the definition as a form of shorthand – in which case there will be very few occasions on which the definition will be useful to him. This biological analogy illustrates the general point that it is not possible to arrive at precise definitions unless the body of knowledge in the relevant field is in an advanced state of organization. Until that stage is reached it is more useful to seek clarity of thought and communication by finding agreement on operational descriptions of phenomena. At least these will assist the student or practitioner in achieving a better orientation in the field of study. But it should still be borne in mind that more precise definitions are valuable when they can be arrived at without distortion or oversimplification of the facts.

The biological analogy can be applied – perhaps with even more relevance – to the field of mental health study and action. There, a more immediate issue is that confusion is resulting not from the inadequacy of practically non-existent available definitions but from the use of confused and conflicting operational descriptions. The Study Group quickly realized that even among its own members the term mental health was being employed, for example, both in the sense of a kind of positive force and as a comprehensive term to embrace a wide spectrum of phenomena of mental health and illness.

The search for improved operational descriptions may be assisted by a brief review of some of the attempts to define mental health that have been published in the literature. It is interesting to find that concern with this subject is very ancient; that, for example, the Hippocratic concept of hysteria was essentially a mental health notion, and that ancient Arabic medical writings record that people could be happier and more effective with symptoms than without.

The whole question is complex in the extreme and much dependent on concepts of normality and abnormality. In his book *The Life of the Genius* Kretschmer asked the question whether a genius should, strictly speaking, be regarded as healthy or unhealthy – and this is only one illustration of a single facet of this subject. On one issue there appears to be a considerable measure of agreement: that mental health is not a static property, but a state that is subject to variation.

In the WFMH Cross-cultural Study No. 2 on 'Mental Health and Value Systems' (41) some of the more recent statements about mental health are discussed, starting with the now famous reference in the Constitution of the World Health Organization, 1947: 'Health is a state of complete physical, mental and social well-being, and not merely the absence of disease or infirmity'. This discussion continued with a reference to the 1948 International Preparatory Commission, which had been concerned with the optimal development of individuals and with the characteristics of the society that promoted such development. In an extended operational description of individual mental health, Soddy (39) stressed, among other points, that the response of the healthy person to life is without strain, that he is capable of both friendship and aggressiveness, that he is consistent and self-reliant but can accept aid, and that his private beliefs are a source of strength to him. Twelve years later, this author himself remarked that this part, at least, of his operational description had been made from a static viewpoint, and that it had not taken variable cultural factors into account. With regard to the latter, it has been pointed out in 'Mental Health and Value Systems' that the quality of consistency would scarcely be valued highly in a society where belief in reincarnation was conventional; as a further example, it should be noted that there are societies in which private beliefs and personal values are a source of strength to the individual only when they are entirely consonant with the values of the community, otherwise they may prove a crippling handicap. It appears that in much that has been written about mental health in recent years a growing realization is being shown that cultural factors enter into mental health phenomena at all levels.

Rümke (38) has added the dimension of the value system to the concept of individual mental health; and O'Doherty (49) has stressed integration of the personality, judgement freed from distortions due to emotional pressure, and consciousness freed from obsession with self. Among other things, he writes, mental health demands good interpersonal relations with oneself, with others, and with God.

A different approach was adopted by Marie Jahoda in compiling the first of a series of monographs published by the Joint Commission on Mental Illness and Health, as part of a national mental health survey in the USA. Using a group of ten consultants, she worked out some of the current concepts of what she termed 'positive mental health'. Her monograph (31) ran to some 22,000 words, which, though quite unacceptable as a definition, may not be excessive as an operational description. Its length is, at least, eloquent testimony to the complexity of her task. Among other contributions, Jahoda introduces two valuable clarifying statements. First: 'Mental health is used to describe a series of services to those sections of the population suffering from some degree of mental disability that the individual, or his associates, believe requires some type of help or intervention.' Second: 'The term "mental health" is also used to describe (i) a state of feeling or being of an individual; (ii) the qualities of a group of almost any size, from family to world, that affect the uniquely human behaviour of its members. Either of these latter uses, describing an emotional or social quality, healthy persons or nations, may have differing degrees of mental health. The orientation of the judge will also affect the judgement of relative merits.'

One of the great bars to an adequate conceptualization of mental health is the habitual use for evaluation by human beings of feeling tone derived from experience of pleasure-pain cycles. Thus, what is memorable to the individual is pleasure or pain experience, but the neutral condition may tend to pass unnoticed and unremembered. A psychiatrist remarked that he had often found it possible to explain to people what health is by saying that when one is in good health one does not think about health, nor, presumably, does one feel anything specific. Health, including mental health, provides a neutral emotional background which enables the individual to experience both pleasurable and painful sensations objectively. The nearest state in sensation that is analogous to mental health is comfort, as distinct from pleasure. Since pain with its attendant anxiety tends to be more memorable than pleasure, ill health and disease, whether physical or mental, may be more memorable than health. Because of this there may be a tendency for absence of pain to be mistaken for comfort, and absence of illness or disease to be mistaken for health.

THE APPROACH TO OPERATIONAL DESCRIPTION

The Study Group recognized that an operational description is an example of understanding by extension on the lines described by Korzybski (662) – the analogical method whereby learning takes place from numerous examples. It has been legitimately stressed by Alan Gregg that an operational description, in addition to referring to the properties of an object, includes what it is not as well as what it forms part of and what it is comprised of. Thus the negative aspects of such descriptions, to which objections are sometimes raised, have a proper part in an operational description in the same way that any processes of identification must include finding out what the object is not, as well as what it is. Thus a complete description of mental health must include mental illness.

Members of the Study Group added a number of thoughts to the discussion of the various attempted definitions in the literature. A psychiatrist with long experience of mental health work in English-speaking countries suggested that the essence of mental health is an attitude of mind that enables the individual to stand up to the difficulties of life, to tackle them without getting unduly anxious, and to be relatively free from obsessional worries and feelings of guilt. He placed emphasis on the development of a sense of responsibility from early childhood, and pointed out that the need for a sense of individual responsibility becomes greater wherever the scope of community responsibility is being enlarged, as in the development of the welfare state. Together with a strong sense of responsibility, the child needs security, and a positive reaction to authority that enables him to be neither overdependent nor with a constant urge to rebel.

One practical difficulty inherent in defining mentally healthy attitudes in terms of responsibility is that of knowing how responsibility can be fostered in young children. A psycho-analyst with wide experience of the mental health of young children commented, as an example, that it is a common characteristic of mothers to regard a toddler child's stubborn behaviour – 'No, no, I'll do it' – as a reprehensible form of obstinacy requiring eradication, and not, as many observers would hold, as the beginnings of development of a healthy independence. One of the problems in fostering a sense of responsibility in a child is to help him to do things for himself, i.e. to take responsibility for the management of his own actions. According to this view, the absence of any sign of stubborn behaviour is unhealthy; parents have little objective cause for satisfaction in having a perfectly compliant and obedient child.

The psycho-analyst suggested that one common practice that operates against the acquisition of a sense of responsibility by young children is that of propping a feeding-bottle by mechanical means.[1] This kind of do-it-yourself activity divorced from the development of any interpersonal relationship can lead only to ego-centred satisfaction-seeking behaviour. It is generally agreed that the child should have ample experience of taking his part in cooperative behaviour in which he or she is given every opportunity to take the initiative compatible with the interests of other members of the family and with safety.

This wider perspective of mental health interest that includes abstract concepts such as that of a sense of responsibility is a prominent example of the significant developments of recent years. Those who are concerned with mental health action have responded to the challenge that has arisen from the identification of social tensions and anxieties which cause suffering and socio-pathological inadequacy, and have sought to enlarge their competence in the face of these largely psychologically determined disturbances. Our knowledge of these matters is still far from complete, both in itself and in its application, and the main aim of mental health action in the next decade should be to gain the competence needed to bring effective help to those who are in need of it, whether individuals or communities or, in the broad perspective, nations.

The perspective of modern mental health concern is wide indeed. It can go deep into the values and desires of individuals and also into the collective ideals and aspirations of groups and communities. Even the aims and motives of nations may come within the ambit – a claim that can be supported by consideration of the perilous situation of the whole world today because the large nations are clinging to power and the newly emerging nations are fast acquiring these menacing values.

In Volume I (Chapter 4) we have discussed a new concept of nationhood that, in our view, is essential for the future of the world. However time-honoured and customary, the aspiration to be a strong national power is no longer compatible with mental

[1] More recently, the Editor read an advertisement for an electrical device to rock the cradle – automation marches on.

health at the international level – indeed it may be argued that it never has been so in the past. Instead of national strength there needs to be substituted the ideal of great nationhood, which would value more highly than any concept of power the ability to live at peace, the capacity to be creative and productive; and would breed citizens who, as individuals, could well withstand the stresses inherent in life without recourse to collective, defensive/aggressive organizations. In short, the goals of mental health action must embrace such concepts as quality of living.

The Study Group agreed that the operational description of mental health should take in these and other more positive factors that go beyond considerations of absence of ill health and of social welfare, but it is important to maintain a balance between the social, medical, and mental aspects. In the words of an educational psychologist, we are working towards 'the newer concept of mental health, itself dependent on a developed capacity to deal with internal conflict and stress in terms of the individual's resources, as opposed to ideas of mental health as absence of conflict or as an "adjustment" by conformity'.

A similar concept was developed by a French-speaking psychiatrist who discussed the meaning of the French phrase *assomption de soi*, which cannot be translated by a simple English synonym. A somewhat wordy English paraphrase might be 'the recognition of oneself for what one is', i.e. both strengths and weaknesses, and the acceptance by the individual of the role in which he is cast by society and by his own abilities (see also 41, 'Mental Health and Value Systems', pp. 131–2).

This part of the discussion reflects an interesting aspect of the modern concept of mental health, for it combines the notions of fulfilment and of realization of the best in oneself, not only deriving the maximum from one's potentialities and life situation, but doing so for ends that are valued as good.

This concept is not mechanistic like that of adaptation, and it contains within itself the idea of an asymptotic aspiration towards perfection. It provides for the full development of the person, in the sense of the term used by Mounier (663), which comprises an ethical content among the various factors that make up the psychological entity of 'personality'.

INDICATORS OF MENTAL HEALTH AND ILL HEALTH

Before attempting to reach an acceptable operational description of mental health, the Study Group wished to broaden the discussion and to consider some of the signs of mental health and ill health in the community. One possible way to determine such indicators of mental health and ill health in the community would be to itemize all the major functions of mental health activities that can be found, to identify the persons involved and their roles, and thence to go on to attempt an operational description of mental health. By adopting this socially based approach, the emphasis would be laid on the mental health of the individual as a function of the person's relationship with the community.

According to an industrial psychologist, mental health action should be conceived in terms of promotion of those social and individual conditions that favour the growth of the creative and cooperative attributes of man. According to this view it is the latter that indicate a state of mental health, but it is irrelevant to attempt to express mental health quantitatively because well-being and the predominance of love over hatred are hardly measurable. Some qualitative indices of a community's level of mental health on the negative side – or its mental ill health – may be looked for in its statistics in respect of mental illness, suicides, alcoholism, drug addiction, delinquency, crime, and public violence; in its divorce, accident, and illegitimacy rates; and in the proportion of its citizens in need of public care.

It was objected from the anthropological point of view that though the above approach might be useful for much of modern, urban, industrialized society, it would have much less value, and no comparative significance, for societies where the social conditions are widely different. It is obvious that in a society in which there is no divorce, or which has different sexual mores in respect of marriage, or where there are very strong religious sanctions against suicide, it would not be possible to use the corresponding criteria as indices of anything other than the existence of cultural differences. No doubt there would be other indices more relevant to the mental health of the culture concerned, but these would need to be worked out. It was suggested, as an example, that hostility or cruelty or despair which, in one society, might both lead to the establishment of and result from the activities of secret police and all that they signify might, in another, contribute to the formation of mobs and determine the type of force used by the society to quell riots; or explain the existence of a large vagrant religious population whose membership is not controlled, such as the Senyussi of India; or have effects in other ways.

To establish any system of indicators, each index must be related specifically to the culture in which it is being applied. The task could be approached by selecting a wide series of possible indicators and studying each one in relation to the culture under consideration. However, since there is so little precise knowledge in this field at the moment, the notion of indices of mental health and ill health is of more significance for the future than for the present. Nevertheless, it is desirable to work towards more effective indicators, not least for the sake of public education in these matters. For example, a large proportion of the news coverage in the press in many countries is devoted to the publicizing of matters that indicate the possibility of a poor quality of mental health among the people referred to – reports on divorce proceedings, alcoholism, murders, or sexual offences. It appears important to us that the proportion of people in the population who realize what is the true significance to the community of such reports should be increased through greater sophistication about mental health matters.

Another way in which the designation of indicators of mental health and ill health can contribute is in the obtaining of support, including financial support, for programmes of mental health activities. It has appeared to be virtually impossible to find support for a programme which defines mental health merely as a state of wellbeing, or by some other so-called 'positive' term. In order to get government money for programmes, it is almost invariably necessary to give quite concrete instances of conditions that need to be corrected. Even with the considerable reservations that must be made, given the present state of knowledge, it still remains a valid objective to work out wherever possible the principal indices for any given community. An example was given from South Africa: whereas an index of illegitimacy would have no meaning in a traditional African society, in the urban communities in South Africa the illegitimacy rates have risen very steeply and today reflect one of the most serious social problems in that country. An index of this order, provided it can be confidently interpreted in its full social context, can be extremely valuable to bring home the need for social action.

It was agreed by the Study Group that though great care must be exercised about making generalizations from any such indices, there are many current circumstances in which the use of reliable indicators could have far-reaching consequences. Experience has shown that mental health action is not likely to be regarded either as realistic or as valuable by the community as a whole unless it is possible to demonstrate the existence of indices of the order which we have discussed. Such indices need to be as specific as possible, and to be developed in terms of both positive and negative criteria with relevance to the individual and to the society. In addition, reliable indices should make it possible to make valid comparisons over time and to assess the extent of change more accurately than can be done at present.

POSITIVE MENTAL HEALTH

The Study Group noted that the term 'positive mental health' has recently come into wide use (31), but considered a number of objections to the introduction at this stage of a concept of polarity or a postulation of a continuum into the attempt to define mental health. Strictly speaking, a positive value can be attached to mental health only if mental health be regarded as neutral, extending on the one side to positive mental health and on the other to negative mental health. This last term might, with justification, be regarded as unhelpful and would need to be replaced by mental ill health or, possibly, mental illness. Either of the latter terms would add semantic complications, involving justifying the notion that illness or ill health forms a single continuum with neutral health and positive health, an exercise which the Study Group regarded more as a speculative manipulation of words than a contribution to present knowledge.

The adoption of mental health as a neutral concept would have additional awkward consequences for WFMH and mental health associations in general, because mental health would no longer be an aspiration or a goal, but merely a statement of a range of interest. It would be necessary to invent some other term to convey the notion of a goal, for it would be difficult to arouse enthusiasm for a national association that was in pursuit of something that was perfectly neutral. The practical issue is that, since mental health and its synonyms are already widely used to express an aspiration, to introduce the term positive mental health only adds to the confusion of thought in an already muddled field.

These objections to the use of the adjective 'positive' in the context of mental health do not apply with equal force to comparative terms, and the Study Group considered whether it might be more legitimate to employ terms relating to a concept of qualitative variations in mental health; specifically, the term 'optimum mental health' to describe 'the best state of mental health that is possible in the particular circumstances' was put forward for discussion.

The concept of optimum mental health was elaborated in functional terms by a psycho-analyst member of the Study Group. He suggested that one of the social functions of mental health is to promote the development, within the capacity of each individual in his culture, of the optimum in human relationships. The key condition here is 'within the capacity of each individual in his culture'. To give a crude example: the criteria for mental health are not the same, in respect of self-identity and so forth, for a three-year-old boy and a thirty-year-old man belonging to the same culture; and in the case of individuals belonging to different cultures, the criteria would vary also according to the different properties of the cultures and the styles of relationship there. An operational definition of mental health could then be made in terms of optimum functioning in relation to the exigencies of life, the stresses in the life situation, the capacities of the individual, and the established criteria of acceptable behaviour in the culture. The indices or criteria of mental health would coincide to some extent with the presumptive norms of behaviour in the society, but for more specific use as practical criteria, these norms would need to be developed to include more of the scientific criteria that are coming to light as knowledge extends.

The Study Group recognized that the meaning of the word 'optimum' is imperfectly understood, being frequently confused with the meaning of 'maximum'. The word optimum embodies the notion of choice and therefore is only properly applicable to the best available. Thus 'optimum' should not be used in an abstract, perfectionist sense but, rather, as the best of a limited range of possible variation. In this sense, a feeble-minded person could be said to have optimum mental health, because although his may not be the best state of mental health that could be conceived, it is the best that is available under the limitations of his intellectual status.

RATIONALIZATION OF TERMINOLOGY

The terminology in the field under discussion is greatly in need of rationalization, which has so far proved very difficult, partly because of the stigma which always attaches to terms that are connected, however remotely or indirectly, with mental disorder; but partly also because of the meanings that have become attached to terms like health and hygiene in their physical sense. 'Health' is often used as if it were almost synonymous with illness, as, for example, in 'health service', which, in some countries, is applied indiscriminately to provisions for the treatment of illness. 'Hygiene' has undergone a similar corruption and now is widely employed in a quite narrow sense, to embrace sanitary measures such as drains and cleanliness, in which usage, ironically, the word 'sanitary' has itself been corrupted.

An attempt by the WHO Expert Committee on Mental Health in 1950 to establish the usage of 'mental health' as a state or condition, and 'mental hygiene' as relating to the techniques and practices used in pursuit of mental health, failed to secure general acceptance. More recently, the term 'positive' has been introduced to fill in the gap in terminology but, as we have discussed above, it has the disadvantage of invoking also the nonsensical concept of negative mental health.

The Study Group agreed to put forward the word 'optimum' as yet another in the series of attempts to rationalize terminology. The main advantages of this term are that it allows for various levels of mental health and also for the specific situation of the individual. Its chief disadvantage is that it may be confused with the 'best' or the 'greatest'.

It may be useful briefly to recapitulate the discussion so far. The term 'mental health', as discussed here, refers to a field of action which is wider than that of a group concerned with the technicalities of the psychodynamics of individuals. (A legitimate comparison might be made with the field of action of a group concerned with the technicalities of psychiatry, or perhaps of education.) The goals of action in the field of mental health are not limited to the attempt to prevent illness, but include those of working towards the optimum, or best possible, mental health of the individual in his or her specific circumstances. These circumstances include age, sex, capacities, culture, social situation, the dimensions of time and locality, and many other relevant factors. The word optimum refers specifically to an individual in given circumstances, or to a group of individuals in a society in given circumstances. It would be valuable to develop a system of indices or indicators of mental health applicable to individuals and, collectively, to societies, and also, if possible, to identify some indices with cross-cultural significance.

The Study Group prefers the use of the concept of optimum mental health to that of positive mental health, being influenced by the implication of the former term as compared with the latter that mental health is itself in part a human value and not a neutral condition. (Elsewhere we have discussed mental health as an instrumental rather than an ultimate value, i.e. a means whereby other values may be obtainable (41).)

We have also discussed elsewhere the view that the mental health worker is committed to an ethical position and that in his work the distinction between what is ethical and what is politic or expedient must be rigorously observed. We are seeking a definition or, as we prefer, an operational description, of mental health, therefore, that is capable of embracing various levels and qualities of mental health, and it is in this complex sense that the term optimum is suggested.

8

An Operational Description

The adoption of a convention about optimum mental health does not itself develop the operational description, and the Study Group considered further aspects of the subject. First, what part does anxiety have in the make-up of the mentally healthy person? It is generally agreed that human life would not have persisted on the earth had human beings not been motivated by anxiety to adapt to circumstances, or even to strive after survival. However, only certain degrees and qualities of anxiety are of biological or survival value, broadly speaking, those that are appropriate to external circumstances and do not persist in the absence of any threat or danger.

To use a simple illustration: where there is a food shortage it would not be mentally healthy, indeed quite the reverse, not to feel anxious about the possibility of starvation, nor would it be mentally healthy to wish to make people free from such anxiety; but in a community where food is plentiful and within reach of all, anxiety about possible starvation is pathological, and requires alleviation in the interests of health.

Second, the concept of mental health with which the Study Group is concerned is relative to time, setting, and circumstance and embraces not only the differences between cultures and social groups within a culture, but also the changes taking place in societies. The concept of relativity in mental health was implicit in the WFMH cross-cultural study 'Mental Health and Value Systems' (41), which had as its subtitle 'An inquiry into the compatibility of mental health concepts with various religions and ideologies'. The practical value of this relative concept is in communication of mental health principles across cultural boundaries, so that relevant techniques of mental health education, training, and so on, developed in one culture can draw with advantage upon the experience of other people. This latter task would be greatly facilitated if agreement could be found on what might be termed a basic core of mental health principles, valid in many cultures and groups.

Third, a psychiatrist advocated that both individual mental health and the mental health of the community be assessed to some extent in quantitative terms. Elsewhere (41) we have taken an analogy from the study of nutrition:

'Nutrition is a state that can be assessed qualitatively, but the success of any attempt at quantification will be dependent upon the amount of available scientific knowledge of the principles that determine a state of good nutrition. What is more, the principles of these basic sciences are, on the whole, exportable across cultural boundaries, and can be applied to the securing of good nutrition just as much in one part of the world as in another, however much food habits may vary.

Therefore, the application of knowledge derived from the appropriate basic sciences can be used to raise standards of nutrition, and to this extent it may be deemed feasible to quantify or measure nutrition.'

It may be asked to what extent can the application of knowledge derived from the appropriate basic sciences in the field of mental health be used to raise the level of mental health? If this could be done, the notion of measurement or quantification of mental health might have some usefulness, but it is clearly a complex concept.

There is no general agreement about how the concept of mental health can be legitimately applied to society, and the Study Group preferred to think of society being conducive to the mental health of its members to a greater or lesser degree or, conversely, to their mental ill health. With this reservation, the quantitative estimation of mental health in society can be approached from another angle. Starting with the premise that there are different levels of mental health of individuals, it might be argued that if the mental health of individuals in the community were to be improved, a general improvement in the level of behaviour in the community would follow, which could be conducive to the mental health of its members to a greater degree than previously. Since there is inevitably some confusion between the ideal and the norm of behaviour of individuals in a society, a rise in levels of individual behaviour might be impossible to identify or measure, but the converse situation – an increased prevalence of regressive behaviour of individuals in a community – might be used to indicate some change in the level of mental health in that society. This indication would be valid only in a society in which there was a certain uniformity of style of behaviour and a recognizable, stable relationship between ideal behaviour and the society's expectations of the individual. The quantitative concept may well have some value for the estimation of ill health even in its present unstandardized state, because a deterioration in individual behaviour – i.e. a falling away from ideals and expectations – in a community might be associated with an increase of mental ill health among its members. It is of interest to note that regression, deterioration, and disintegration of individual behaviour, and breakdown of interpersonal relationships are commonly cited as evidence of community mental ill health.

The Study Group thought that it was a legitimate conclusion that anything that can be done to raise the capacity of the individual to come to terms with himself and to achieve the full realization of his own potential; and, conversely, anything that can be done to reduce the negative aspects of individual behaviour, could contribute positively to mental health in the community.

However, it needs to be recognized that it is possible for individuals to get caught up in developments and social processes which may lead them into regressive behaviour, although they themselves might be regarded, with justice, as mentally healthy individuals. For example, an individual who has been brought up remote from other communities of different race or colour can hold firmly to discriminatory attitudes because of lifelong exposure to the unchallenged assumptions of his own group, which are the result of a complete absence of relationship with other groups. It could hardly be said that a prejudice under such conditions would necessarily be mentally unhealthy; but if it should persist after a relationship has been established with another group, the question of a mentally unhealthy attitude would arise.

MENTAL HEALTH CONCEPTS
AND EDUCATIONAL THOUGHT

In a working paper, Morris drew attention to the affinities between mental health concepts and modern teaching on child development. He remarked:

'. . . accepted doctrines among educators emphasize the growth of the child as a whole, the close interrelation of maturation and nurture, the importance of readiness, of developmental sequences, of personally meaningful activity, of play and creative expression, of individual differences in capacities, temperaments, and interests and individually adjusted goals in learning. Stress is on development from within, the unfolding of powers under the stimulation, support, and guidance of teachers. School is thought of as offering community life in miniature and in many ways compensating for deficiencies in home environment.

There is need to supplement and deepen these concepts from two other main sources which are not yet so widely accepted among educators:

Psychodynamic concepts – for example, the power and complexity of emotional drives, particularly love, hate, and fear; the basic need for love and security in coming to terms with destructive impulses and in forming non-oppressive internal controls; the ubiquitous character of unconscious mental functioning and its relation to conscious functioning; the internal sources of conflict and their interaction with external ones; the power and importance of phantasy, and the need for creative activity in coming to terms with feeling and impulse and in giving form and direction to the mastering of the external world; defensive manoeuvres and adjustments; importance of ego strength for stability of personality; identification and the patterning of relationships in the contexts of family and later environments; dependence and independence; the relation between external and internal authority; the search for personal identity; personality as a more or less strongly integrated dynamic structure; the dynamic role of the teacher in interpersonal relations (instead of being merely a neutral guide) and in particular in the dynamics of the class group; and the newer concept of mental health itself as dependent on a developed capacity to deal with internal conflict and stress in terms of the individual's resources, as opposed to ideas of mental health as absence of conflict or as "adjustment" by conformity. Thus deepened, the psychology of development becomes a formidable problem in the training of teachers.

Cross-cultural and subcultural studies – the general influence of these in calling attention to the errors of ethnocentric thinking and in emphasizing the differences of social and educational traditions, developmental norms and value systems between cultures and within the same culture, thus strengthening understanding of the immense variety of expression of our common humanity and deepening the capacity to discern and respect "the other".'

OPERATIONAL DESCRIPTION OF MENTAL HEALTH

Two major lines of approach have been considered. The first is by the extension of the concept of the social role of mental health. In other words, the social implications of action for mental health in the community might give a lead towards a deeper philosophical understanding of mental health, and at the same time might enable further definition, coordination, and integration of planning of mental health societies.

The second approach to an operational description is to regard mental health as an abstract end-result of numerous specific contributing factors. A psychiatrist gave an illustration from the history of the classical methods of teaching medical students. At one time neurotic illness was thought to be a result of a defect of the will, so that it was logical to treat neurosis by exhorting the patient to mobilize 'will-power'. It is now recognized that whatever is meant by will-power is not a separable faculty of the mind, but, rather, a stream of mental activity which can reach its fullest development only when mental activity as a whole is functioning in an integrated and (relatively) unimpaired way. Thus both will-power and the capacity to mobilize it are functions of the mentally healthy mind, and the therapist's exhortation, if it has any effect at all, can result only in increasing the amount of emotional conflict in the patient's mind.

Another illustration can be taken from the interaction within organized groups, in this instance from military psychiatry: a psychiatrist remarked that experience during World War II had shown that 'good morale' is not a separate entity obtainable by intensive drill, ruthless inspections, 'pep talks', or whatever the commanders may happen to believe in, but a sort of 'bloom' on the fruit of a good military unit. This good morale might be regarded as a holistic description of the near-perfection of its integrated, efficient, adaptable, and confident function, and might be as near to a description of optimum group mental health as one could expect to get.

One constant difficulty about the use of abstractions taken from operational descriptions is that attention may get focused on the abstraction itself, which then becomes the subject of attempts to define more narrowly. This appears to have happened in a great deal of thinking about mental health, as the many discussions about such matters as morale and will-power have shown. On the other hand, and at the other extreme, as an example of the more pragmatic operational approach of the social role of mental health, Binet is reported to have replied to a question as to what intelligence is: 'This is what my test is measuring, and if you want to know what intelligence is you must take my test.' Another remark in the same vein, attributed to Binet, was that the tests measured the score that children got on the tests. The excessive caution of the latter remark is hardly likely to clarify the operational description of mental health, but there is a great deal to be said in favour of adopting with moderation the pragmatic descriptive approach, and of studying closely the activities that are undertaken in the name of mental health. The lack of a satisfactory definition of intelligence has not sterilized psychology, and we have no reason to suppose that a similar lack of definition in the case of mental health will necessarily be harmful to the latter.

It is a commonplace to attack the widespread loose tendency to describe mental health in terms of mental ill health, but this criticism carries weight only so long as there is an absence of any more positive operational description of mental health. The descriptive terms need to cover a wide range of individual and social developmental, behavioural, and ethical phenomena, and to maintain a balance between positive and negative elements. This applies to any operational description, and not less to pragmatic description than to that of abstract quality.

It may legitimately be argued that the application to mental health of the analogy taken above from intelligence-testing carries the pragmatic approach too far. It may be agreed that operational techniques are scientifically valid only if there is some certainty about what the operation is yielding. In other words, in the case of intelligence tests, do the tests in fact give the kind of information that is being looked for? However great their contribution, the tests have not been sufficient in themselves to evaluate intelligence, and it is probable that every psychologist working in the cognitive field has some concept of the appraisal of intelligence that does not depend on the tests that have been devised. But the tests are undoubtedly helpful, and it may be inferred that the next most useful stage in developing the operational description of mental health would be to study the significance of those component parts of the description for which there are well-established precedents in the contributing professional fields.

No doubt past attempts at the operational description of mental health have been weaker on the positive side; this may have been the effect of traditional methods of teaching by demonstrating sickness, referred to above. We have discussed elsewhere the apparent difficulty in this field of being explicit about positive values – about what is good. Somehow, shyness or diffidence comes over the mental health worker when it is suggested that he or she is attempting to do good and yet, in our view at least, every mental health worker is *ipso facto* committed to an ethic.

A number of attempts have been made to introduce positive descriptive terms such as creativity, delight, sharing delight, or fulfilment. It is often easy to recognize in certain people a combination of qualities that enables them not only to live emotionally satisfying and full lives, but to communicate this fact by the atmosphere that surrounds them. It may be that closer investigation of this phenomenon would illuminate some of the obscurities in the operational description of mental health.

An operational description rather than a definition of mental health would be of particular advantage for the educational or propaganda aspects of mental health work. We have discussed above some of the emotionally determined attitudes of ordinary people which can complicate mental health work, and the tendency for a stigma to become attached to all terms that are employed in this field. The devaluation of the term mental health itself has been a major reason for the search for more positive synonyms. The stigma is itself hardly predictable; for example, it was agreed at the Study Group meeting that in some English-speaking countries the use of the term 'emotional health' has, surprisingly, proved more effective in propaganda work than the term mental health. It appears to elicit a more positive response, and people are more inclined to apply it to themselves, whereas the term mental health is more often applied to the mentally ill.

The precise ways in which the current concept of mental health can best be projected into the understanding of the general population were the subject of considerable discussion. The need for the use of terms more specific than 'positive mental health' and 'making well people better' was emphasized. A psychiatrist with experience of public health work observed that legislators can easily understand the concept of preventing disease, provided it is employed strictly in a specific sense, but that even the term 'prevention' used in a general way is difficult to project. It is not easy, to say the least, to show what has to be prevented, once the cruder sources of stress and strain in society have been removed. The psychiatrist added that, in the American view, laughing children and happiness are normal parts of life and they should not need a specific programme, under whatever name, for their promotion.

A psychiatrist in the intergovernmental field of work did not agree that there was a necessary contradiction between a positive mental health programme and one that sets out to minimize mental illness. A sound objective is the formation in the public mind of an image of mental health that includes both positive and negative aspects, some of which can be promoted best by the use of mass media and advertising, others by education, feedback, and more personal methods.

There is considerable preoccupation in mental health circles with the question of influencing the legislator, so that new laws and social practices can be introduced in the interests of mental health. On the other hand, some people question whether it is an essential part of preventive mental health work to project a new image of optimum mental health onto the legislator; and whether it might not be better to concentrate first on the improvement of mental hospitals. Hospitals can be improved by legislation, to some extent, but not unless the legislators understand how bad the hospitals are now. It is of interest to note that it is current practice in the Soviet Union for whatever concept exists there of optimum mental health to be put forward, not by the mental health experts, but by the government department concerned with cultural matters. This arrangement reflects the attitude that the population itself is regarded as the expert on mental health, and the technicians as being concerned only with the illness aspects. Since it is generally agreed that mental health in the full sense of the term cannot be promoted solely by legislation, the

Study Group accepted in principle that those promoting mental health in the community should concern themselves with legislators only in respect of the treatment of mental illness and related matters; but the ramifications of the role of the technician are another matter altogether, upon which little agreement with the implied Russian view seems to exist.

An African psychiatrist thought that in many countries, and particularly those that are newly emerging, it is impossible to draw any distinction between the prevention of illness and the promotion of the so-called more positive aspects of mental health. In all health education, he said, the primary consideration is the level and nature of understanding of the public and how the latter may be motivated. Therefore the material must be presented in terms of concrete situations that people can understand. In much of the world it is virtually impossible at the present time to speak in terms of positive mental health. On the contrary, the starting-point has to be the prevention of illness by improving the efficiency of therapeutic methods, minimizing the harm done by ill people in the population, and correcting tendencies and practices known to foster illness, whether in the family, in educational processes, or in human relations at large. Perhaps the first essential is to demonstrate how current factual knowledge can best be applied to situations which the people can recognize. This has brought the discussion back to the starting-point – the birth of mental health work.

THE WIDENING CONCEPT OF MENTAL HEALTH

We have traced the development of the concept of mental health from its origins in the early attempts to improve the quality of care and treatment of mental disorder, to the more modern multi-disciplinary action that takes place on a wide social field, and nowadays is reaching out to involve even the aspirations of nations in the modern world. We have stressed the modern ideal of great nationhood, by which mankind as a whole may find satisfaction in quality of living, and we have stated our conviction that this can be a realizable ideal, with the rider that unless significant progress is made towards the attainment of this ideal, the world will continue to be in dire peril.

Much of the recent widening of the mental health horizon has been due to the involvement of professional disciplines that have hitherto been engaged solely on curative work in studying problems of human relationships, both in normal social situations and under conditions of external stress. We have referred to the work of psychiatrists and psychologists in the armies of various countries in World War II, as a result of which a great deal has been learnt about human reactions under stress and about group morale. The integrated interdisciplinary approach of psychiatrists, psychologists, sociologists, anthropologists, and so on, has been developed, and similar techniques have been applied to industrial and social problems in many countries. In fact, the professions concerned have moved a long way from their former preoccupations with phenomenological descriptions and pathology in their specific fields, to their current concern with questions of human relationships in many different kinds of situation.

The widening of scope and the involvement of many professional disciplines in mental health work have caused a certain diffuseness, if not confusion, of aim, and in some ways have also led to an unconstructive overlap of professional fields. The protagonists of the wider concept of mental health have tended to make the assumption that a kind of continuum exists, from mental illness at one extreme, through health regarded as an absence of mental illness, to, at the other extreme, the optimum development of the human being as a member of the human species. The acceptance of the whole spectrum as the proper field of mental health presents an impossible task, unless the specific concerns within it are narrowed. Since the end of World War II mental health workers have tended increasingly to include almost every human interest and activity within their scope, from questions of universal peace to the best types of housing. There has been a great deal of overlap between the fields of action of mental health and those of public health, education, home economics, urban planning, and technical-assistance programmes – to name only a few. Although some overlap is useful and, in fact, essential for interdisciplinary activity, unless each professional discipline is clear about respective areas of professional competence and the ways in which overlap can be made constructive, the whole situation becomes confused, and the various professions will tend to compete with rather than complement each other.

For example, mental health workers dealing with the individual commonly draw attention to the effects of bad housing on family relationships in particular cases or in general, but housing is not really their business. Mental health workers are also interested in the effects of malnutrition, especially when it impairs mental functioning or causes mental disease, but they are not primarily concerned with nutrition as such. Similarly, the problems of war, peace, and survival as such are not primarily their business, but mental health workers may have a great deal to contribute about the attitudes of individuals to these questions, the kinds of conditions that may change people's attitudes, and the extent to which individual reactions affect community behaviour, in both its positive and its negative aspects.

The Study Group considered that extreme attitudes towards these problems – complacency on the one hand and apathy or indifference on the other – could be regarded as coming directly within the field of interest of mental health. Our main concern is with the facilitation of human function and our interest lies more in the origin and significance of human behaviour than in its manifest content. Thus the mental health worker is concerned not so much with the fact that the contemporary world is in danger as with the mental health of the individual who consciously recognizes that the world is in danger, and, much more important, with the question of making an effort, and what kind of effort, to save the world.

In Volume I of this report, in a review of trends over the period 1948 to 1961, it was observed that whereas the International Preparatory Commission of 1948 took as its province the question of world citizenship, the 1961 Study Group was more occupied with questions of attitudes towards interdependence and towards consciousness of the world network of relationships, and with the issues of survival and destruction that confront us. The Study Group concluded that the best contribution of mental health to the solution of these vital issues would be greater study of the mental health aspects of the complex problems involved.

THE PROFESSIONS ENGAGED IN MENTAL HEALTH WORK

One practical implication of the widening of the mental health concept is the broadening of the range of professions that are involved in mental health work. If the field of mental health extends all the way from the prevention of mental illness to the enhancement of full human potentiality, the professions concerned will include those of education, vocational counselling, paediatrics, and many others, no less than psychiatry, psychology, and sociology. This is an extension of the principle already widely accepted that the infant welfare or well-baby clinic is the place not only where the mother is taught to recognize the signs of illness but where she also learns to bring up healthy babies.

The main difficulty about enumerating the professions now involved is that, as has been pointed out, almost everyone who deals with people may be involved in some mental health problem. Thus it is frequently claimed that such-and-such a profession is omitted from consideration. Perhaps the commonest complaints about professions left out of discussions on mental health work refer to general medical practitioners and nurses.

After considerable deliberation, the Study Group was in agreement that the question had not been resolved, whether it was more useful to regard certain professions as primary mental health professions or to regard everyone who has professional dealings with human beings as potentially working in the mental health field. To designate a range of allegedly more specific mental health professions might lead to increased rigidity and competition in the field, and it might be preferable to keep mental health work open to a wide range of people. In this field in particular the maintenance of old hierarchies of professional importance and the establishment of new ones should be avoided. Such an attitude towards professional involvement is especially valuable in relation to the question of community mental health or, as we have preferred to express it, what it is in a society that is conducive to the mental health of individuals. An alternative way of expressing this concept would be to refer to those qualities of a group that affect the uniquely human behaviour of its members. Inasmuch as a wide range of professional people may contribute to the qualities of a group in the sense that we advocate, they may equally contribute to the mental health of the society. This attitude towards professional roles is consonant with the operational description of mental health as made up of the overall functioning of many interacting factors not only in different degrees but also in different combinations or qualities.

A Group member summed up this discussion with the remark that two fundamental questions are being asked: What is it that unites the professions in this field? And what is it that distinguishes them from each other in terms of particular competence? In principle, the answer to the first question – what unites the professions – might be summarized as a concern for human welfare; and this might form a continuum of concern, from what might be done about crippling illness to how to help the individual to live an effective, creative, and happy life.

What distinguishes the professions from each other is the manner in which they are concerned. The educator, for example, is not concerned in the same way and to the same extent as the psychiatrist in cases of crippling illness, and, on his part, the psychiatrist is not so intimately concerned as the educator with the great majority of children, in helping them to grow up to live happy, effective, and creative lives. Each profession can, however, contribute positively to the other's competence.

Reflecting on the discussion of the concept of mental health from an Asian viewpoint, a psychiatrist remarked that no Chinese expression for positive mental health had yet appeared, and he suggested that this could be for the practical reason that the Chinese people were perhaps more realistic in their aims and preoccupied with the immediate task. This observation, he said, was not put forward in any spirit of opposition to the idea of a mental health 'movement', which, although many object to the use of the word 'movement', might be taken to indicate the existence of long-range goals, including what is meant by so-called positive mental health. It might be claimed with justification that these long-range goals are common to all endeavour for human welfare, and are aimed at by educationists, psychological scientists, social workers, and all the other professions that, directly and indirectly, are engaged in this work.

Although the individual professional person may legitimately claim a concern with these ultimate goals, he may well feel that discussion of the goals themselves is more within the competence of the philosophers. However, many mental health workers feel that they have a duty to share in the pursuit of these ideals without claiming competence to teach others to join in the common aim. This shared pursuit of ideals involves working with others who are interested and who have competences of various sorts, and planning together how each can best contribute from his own field of skill to the enrichment of the common fund of knowledge.

The Asian psychiatrist in the Study Group described a discussion of a proposed Chinese translation of *Mental Health and World Citizenship* (12) with educationists and philosophers well versed in Confucian writings. Although the latter thought that the subject-matter of the book had been dealt with 2,000 years ago by Confucius, and were not convinced that the so-called mental health disciplines were competent to operate in this field of ideas, it was still found possible to work together to contribute to the general pool of knowledge, drawing on the insights gained in the examination of human subjects to further understanding of the psychodynamics of human relationships, and making use of the skills of the social sciences.

The Study Group concluded its examination of the question of the conceptualization of mental health by reiterating its conviction that all those who are interested in mental health can contribute to the common aim of human welfare but that each contribution must be made at a realistic level. The role of the individual professional worker is to operate within his own recognized field of competence, in a spirit of willingness to reach out towards the frontiers of knowledge which relate him to members of the other professions concerned.

PART THREE

Professional Training and Public Education

9
Professional Training in Mental Health Subjects

In the postwar years there has been increasing activity as regards training in mental health subjects – for specialists in psychiatry and also for personnel in other branches of medicine and in other professions whose work involves close contact with people. But it is still the case that in no country do the training arrangements in any branch of mental health work even remotely approach adequacy. In many parts of the world training facilities in this field are virtually non-existent.

It is clearly impossible to arrive at any generalization as to basic principles that might be universally applicable to the training of any of these groups. In his preparatory work for the International Study Group, Ahrenfeldt pointed out that even in those countries where mental health training facilities are well organized and involve relatively large numbers of people, there is frequently great variation in the standard and range of the training provided. The field is widely underdeveloped and it is only rarely that training in mental health principles is available for professional people other than psychiatrists.

In this chapter we make no more than a passing reference to the main features of the training of those professions that are most closely engaged in mental health work. The discussion is concentrated on some of the more interesting new developments in the common training of members of professions less centrally concerned with the mental health field, who might, nevertheless, be expected to find an understanding of mental health principles of particular value in the pursuance of their calling.

TRAINING OF PSYCHIATRISTS IN MENTAL HEALTH WORK
With the vast expansion of psychiatric work outside the walls of

161

the mental hospital, the role of the psychiatrist in the community is changing, and his training requirements are changing too. In most parts of the world up to the end of World War II, the great weight of psychiatric training had been undertaken on an in-service basis in hospitals, although various forms of training analysis had been gaining ground. Since that time, far more attention has been paid in many countries to the preparation of the psychiatrist for various types of work in the community setting: in conjunction with community agencies, in a counselling role with professional workers dealing with people, in public administration, and in public health. Current therapeutic emphases are changing, so that the psychiatrist now must be equipped not only to undertake group therapy himself and to operate in the atmosphere of a therapeutic community, but also to give training in appropriate therapeutic roles to other professional personnel, such as general practitioners, public health doctors and nurses, prison officials, educators, and so on.

The training of the psychiatrist was discussed in the published report (603) of the conference on psychiatric education held at Cornell University in 1952. More recent years have seen a great increase in the number of university departments devoted to psychiatry, with a steady growth in the number of professorial chairs. There has been a serious lag – in fact, with very few exceptions, no progress at all – in the development of university departments of child psychiatry.

MENTAL HEALTH TRAINING OF THE MEDICAL
UNDERGRADUATE

Progress in this field continues to be extraordinarily patchy. There are still a large number of countries where even the basic general training needs of medical personnel are not adequately met by the medical schools, either because of a shortage of teachers or because of the range and quality of the teaching. In no country can it be claimed that psychiatry has its proper share of the curriculum as an undergraduate subject, and in many countries the teaching of psychiatry is ignored in medical schools. The argument that is most commonly advanced in opposition to increasing psychiatric time in the medical curriculum is that the curriculum is already overloaded. There appears to be a vicious circle here, in that the senior staffs of medical schools are themselves still largely ignorant of, and sometimes hostile to what they know about, the significance of psychiatry and modern mental health principles, and therefore do not encourage the expansion of undergraduate teaching in this field. It is only fair to mention, though, that in a number of countries, particularly in the United States, there is evidence of a stimulating new approach to the problem of teaching medical students in these subjects (586, 587, 593). The teaching of psychiatry through films and television (621, 622) is increasingly proving its value.

TRAINING OF MEDICAL GRADUATES IN MENTAL HEALTH
The training of general practitioners in psychotherapy in the United Kingdom was discussed in an article by Balint (606). This is a relatively new move, which deserves close attention. In the United States the training of public health doctors as community mental health specialists has been undertaken at Harvard University (610). In the United Kingdom an initiative by the Tavistock Clinic, London, has resulted in the widespread adoption of programmes for the group training of public health doctors and nurses, together with psychiatrists and psychiatric social workers. A relatively new technique, known as a 'demonstration clinic', has been developed in New York (601).

OTHER PROFESSIONS WORKING DIRECTLY
IN THE MENTAL HEALTH FIELD
In 1961 it was still true that only in fairly exceptional or localized instances were any classes of medical (non-psychiatric) or non-medical professional personnel in the mental health field receiving any kind of training in mental health principles, though a number of professions have extended their training into some areas of psychiatry and clinical psychology.

The nearest to a formal type of mental health training for a particular profession has been reached in the United States, in the training of psychiatric social workers. As pioneered in the second decade of the century, it consisted of a certain constellation of training and experience which has been followed, more or less closely, though with some modifications, in its spread during the third decade to the United Kingdom and a few other countries. It is probably true to say that during the third and fourth decades of this century psychiatric social workers were, on the whole, more highly trained in mental health subjects than were psychiatrists. It is, however, difficult to compare many areas of the world in respect of this relatively new profession because the designation 'psychiatric social worker' is applied to a variety of types of worker in the field of mental disorders. Thus in some countries those who are working in the field under this name may be without the casework and preventive skills that have been aimed at in the prescribed training of psychiatric social workers, and in not a few countries they may be without any formal training.

The training of psychiatric social workers is nowhere regarded as ideal, being in most countries too short for maximum effectiveness, and presenting the trainee with a difficult choice of orientation between social work, on the one hand, and psychiatry, on the other. The more specifically mental health aspects of the training of psychiatric social workers were the subject of recommendations by the American Association of Psychiatric Social Workers in 1950 (614), and by a Ministry of Health Committee on the future of the social services in the mental health services in the United Kingdom in 1951 (152); but progress in this area remains disappointingly slow.

In the field of nursing training there have been two major trends in the last decade or so: the first is a movement in a number of countries towards raising the standards of technical training of psychiatric nurses in order to make them more on a par, professionally, with general nurses. Traditions in this respect vary widely, but in many countries it has been the practice to draw upon students of lower educational standard for a restricted field of psychiatric nursing. In the United States, where nursing staffing problems have been acute in the last decade, there have been some moves towards a greater specialization of nurses, including psychiatric nurses, compensated for, to some extent, by the introduction of less skilled nursing aides into hospitals. The second general trend has been to incorporate the teaching of principles of mental health and human relations in the training of general nurses. Recommendations were made on this point by an Expert Committee of WHO in 1956 (620), but there are very few places in which they have been implemented on anything more than a strictly local scale, depending upon individual initiative.

The training of professional workers for child guidance units has been discussed by Buckle and Lebovici (283). In this area, too, comparisons between countries are hard to make because there are many different conceptions of the functions of the child guidance worker, and therefore many different views on what kind of training is most appropriate. Some realignments of professional function are taking place here, including the greater involvement of public health personnel, doctors, and nurses in the work of child guidance clinics, and the creation of another relatively new profession – that of clinical psychology – which is the clinical analogue of the profession of educational psychology in relation to problems of education.

The emerging profession of clinical psychology is regarded by many people as a logical outcome of the developments in psychometry that have taken place in the last few decades, tending to make the clinical psychologist more than a diagnostic technician, important though his role has been in introducing more precise and comparable diagnostic methods into child psychiatry. There is less general acceptance for the increasing involvement of the clinical psychologist in the process of making a diagnosis and, in some places, in therapy. In view of the world-wide shortage of professional personnel of all classes in mental health work, it is inevitable that those who are available should be called upon to undertake a wider range of functions than they may be professionally prepared for. In some countries this situation is creating difficulties of cooperation between those who hold a qualification in psychological medicine and psychologists who are not medically qualified.

THE CONTRIBUTIONS OF THE VARIOUS PROFESSIONS

In most countries, however, the real points at issue are quite other than which profession has most right to work in which field. Given the general shortage of trained personnel and the increasing demand, it would be more realistic, almost everywhere, to make an appreciation of the qualities of the various professions working in their different ways within the mental health field, and to consider how the whole field could be best covered.

During the course of discussion at the Study Group it was estimated that in some countries as many as forty different kinds of personnel might be occupationally involved, more or less directly, in some activity of significance to mental health. This formidable figure includes all those whose work affects the life of ordinary people, for example: medical, paramedical, and public health personnel; those who work for religious, social, charitable, educational, workers', legal, and police agencies; promoters of youth organizations; many government and local government officials; and the vast army of those who spend their working hours making house-to-house visits – debt-collecting, insurance-collecting and -selling, even the purveyors of consumer goods on delayed-payment plans and the pedlars of lottery tickets! While recognizing that we are not at present in a position to influence those whose house-to-house calling is motivated by the desire for commercial gain, the Study Group considered that we have a clear duty to promote better standards of mental health training among those professionally engaged in dealing with people, with their daily lives and problems. One preliminary question is: what aspects of training can be common to these professions, and where is specialization appropriate?

It is clear that, in different countries, workers with different titles and training backgrounds are performing essentially similar functions. Work practices and divisions tend to evolve by historical accident or incident, and it is not necessarily the most suitable type of worker who becomes involved, at least in the earlier stages of development.

It would be useful to make a comparative transnational survey in a number of countries of who does what, and how and where, in the mental health field generally. This would be a complex undertaking, and although the absence of established criteria of either success or failure would be a difficulty in the interpretation of the data, the information gained could hardly fail to provide a better basis for the planning of training programmes than conjecture and uncontrolled imitation, which often determine new action at the present time.

The Study Group was concerned with the quality of professional work undertaken in the fields of mental health and human welfare generally. In every country in which there are openings for professional work in these fields the demand for skilled personnel exceeds the available supply; consequently, the gap tends to be filled partly by untrained people of goodwill motivated by ideals of service, but also by the modern counterpart of the mediaeval mountebank and charlatan – the patent-medicine sellers, the mind developers and memory trainers, and those who still practise on the fringes of medicine and magic.

What may be more inimical to the eventual proper development of scientific services are the efforts of people with a pseudo- or para-scientific form of training, e.g. chiropractors, scientologists, christian scientists, herbalists, phrenologists, hypnologists, those who give public demonstrations, and those who apply the principles of moral rearmament as a simple cure-all. These people operate with various degrees of systematization and training. It was the Study Group's view that though it is necessary to make clear what are regarded as minimal qualifications and training for undertaking mental health work, essentially it is the quality of the service provided that must influence the public's choice between mental health workers and others who claim these areas as their province.

The academic disciplines are not sufficient in themselves for the training of workers in the mental health field, especially in the professional functions of psychotherapy and counselling. Experience indicates that skill in psychotherapy can be gained only by practice under the supervision of an experienced therapist; and counselling, which involves far more than the mere handing-out of advice, and indeed is useless without the acceptance of the counsel by the patient, depends for its success on skill of communication, which, again, cannot be acquired merely by academic means. Where professional personnel are in short supply, counselling is probably the most economical and effective form of mental health activity, but it is liable to be more or less stultified when not accompanied by the necessary communication skills.

Mental health problems present remarkably varied forms in different cultures, and it appeared to the Study Group that the qualifications of the professional people concerned may need to differ accordingly. For example, the character of the prevailing religion in the community may be one determinant of what type of person is best suited to undertake mental health work there. In Christian and Islamic cultures the role of the priest or minister of religion is obviously a powerful influence in this connexion, but in the case of religions that are not based on revelation, e.g. Buddhism and Hinduism, the priest's role in mental health work appears to have been less prominent hitherto.

Any attempt to formulate general principles of training has to contend with widely different methods of organizing university training. For example, in some countries universities are independent of government control, whereas in others they are completely dependent upon it, and in yet others partially dependent; again, in some countries universities undertake practical technological training, and in others they are not involved in this way.

We have noted some of the differences that have to be taken into account in considering the subject of training; there are also concerns in common, one of the chief being a widespread realization of the need to revise current concepts of illness. In most countries nosological concepts have been developed from the models of bodily or somatic illness, and they often have little relevance to modern psychological thought. For instance, it may be questioned whether it is valid to make a clear distinction between neurosis and psychosis. It has long been recognized that neither term represents a nosological entity, but that each covers a number of complex patterns of symptoms. A psychiatrist member of the Study Group suggested that it might be more useful to classify mental disorders in terms of urgency, seriousness, and danger involved. How this classification might cut across existing nosological patterns can be seen in the following examples: chronic insanity is often neither urgent nor dangerous, but in terms of prognosis it is usually serious; social neurosis could also be serious, but it would be unlikely to be either urgent or dangerous unless it affected a key figure in the community; melancholia might not be serious in terms of prognosis, especially when effective treatment is available, but it is commonly both urgent and dangerous; acute schizophrenia is probably an urgent problem, commonly but not necessarily serious, and rarely dangerous.

One weakness of professional training for work in this field is the lack of any attempt to impart to those who are most closely concerned with mental health action and the human behavioural sciences some awareness of the insights of the professions less directly involved. To create wider understanding at this level would be an educational ideal in tune with the spirit of the age, encouraging the current trend for the professions to enter each other's worlds, to make more use of each other's languages, and to work with each other's professional insights. To what extent such objectives are practicable could be determined only by further study. As one member of the Study Group pointed out, they imply in some degree a return to the mediaeval notion of the *studium generale*.

PROFESSIONAL ROLES
Prevalent attitudes and trends in respect of professional roles need to be re-examined. It appears to be a universal development that as functions become differentiated in a society each particular

role tends to become the exclusive field of one occupational category, and occupational restrictive and defensive attitudes and practices proliferate. As it has become increasingly professionalized the field of human welfare has proved no exception; for example, in the promotion of programmes for the mental health education of ministers of religion, it is common to meet objections to the acquisition of clinical skills by ministers on the grounds that they would thereby become 'amateur psychiatrists'. A similar objection is often made to the training of social workers in dynamic principles, lest they should become 'amateur psychoanalysts'. The Study Group, though by no means explicit and united in any view to the contrary was, on the whole, more concerned with getting some reversal of these attitudes. It was felt that present conditions would be better served by less rather than more definition of professional frontiers, and by a freer passage of skills and insights from one profession to another.

We would advocate an extensive review of professional roles in the light of the various specific functions that are necessary in the community. For example, in a society where one of the revealed religions is the prevailing one, it is usual for the priest or minister to be closely associated with the critical points of life – birth, confirmation or other initiation ceremonies, marriage, serious illness, death – and any system of mental health education or social programme planning that leaves out the priest will not be realistically based in that society. In this context, the real objective of helping the priest to gain insights from mental health disciplines is not that he shall function, perhaps inadequately, as a psychiatrist, but that he shall function more adequately as a priest. Set out in words this may appear a very obvious conclusion, but it is remarkable to what an extent such issues can be obscured by feelings of professional exclusiveness.

The suggestion that insights should be more freely exchanged between professions is very different from the promotion of uniformity of function, with which it is often confused by its opponents. The Study Group considered that one of the most significant advantages of more completely shared insights would be, far from the promotion of uniformity, that professional differentiation of function could be defined more clearly and on much more rational grounds, with a greater likelihood of acceptance by the professions concerned. An improved interprofessional exchange would improve the cooperation of certain of the non-medical professions not only in the early detection of illness and in prevention, but also, where appropriate, in therapy. Nevertheless, distinctions between professional functions must be maintained: while, for example, ministers of religion and educationists undoubtedly have important roles in the early detection and prevention of illness, their own professions demand more from them than this. The teacher is concerned with all-round healthy development in the mental field even more than with the prevention of disorder; and the same is true, in a different context, of the minister of religion.

On the whole the Study Group was dissatisfied with attempts that have been made to distinguish professional roles by means of terms such as normal and abnormal, or diagnosis and therapy, as commonly found among psychiatrists and non-medical psychologists respectively. The Study Group took the view that such distinctions are often no more than artificial, and sometimes impossible to make. Even in the case of a single profession individuals have different levels of competence in different aspects: for example, a psychiatrist might be very able in the prevention of mental illness through skill in diagnosis, but have little competence in the treatment of schizophrenia, and therefore he would not conform to a common stereotype.

CORE CURRICULUM

This discussion led the Study Group to an apparently inescapable conclusion that the legitimate roles of the various professions and the trainings needed to support these roles are so intermingled that the idea of a basic 'core curriculum' should receive far more attention than it has done hitherto. A fundamental feature common to all the professions under consideration is interpersonal relationships – whether they are termed doctor–patient, social worker–client, or priest–parishioner relationships. In this area it would appear that a core curriculum could make a great contribution to training; and in support of this view it is reported from many places that there is an increasing demand for more adequate training in the understanding of the concepts of psychiatry and dynamic psychology in the education programmes of numerous professional groups whose work brings them into close contact with people. Those aspects of training in which the issues involved are interpersonal relationships and the effect of one person on another cannot be effectively handled by didactic methods, and are very expensive both in time and in training personnel.

The Group was in agreement that, though a number of professions recognize their training need in this connexion, and the case of the clergy has already been stressed, the key people at the present time are those who are responsible for the training of teachers, with particular reference to the interaction of psychology and educational principles. Unless trainers of teachers gain professional competence in respect of interpersonal relations and in the principles of mental development and of psychopathology, it is hardly likely that any great advances can be made in preventive mental hygiene programmes in schools.

One useful method of moving towards a core curriculum is by instituting a joint training programme for students of two or more professions, in certain aspects of their course. There have been many examples in recent years of the interprofessional training of students in clinical subjects. A growing practice is to demonstrate doctor–patient or social worker–client interaction before a one-way screen which is watched by students of various disciplines, who then discuss afterwards with the demonstrator what they have witnessed. This practice has been frowned upon by some people, mainly those unfamiliar with the needs and conditions of clinical training, on the ground of professional ethics. Others have found that, provided they are careful to secure the informed assent of the patient or client, and provided the students are responsibly alive to the confidential nature of the proceedings, as all students of a clinical discipline must be, no difficulties arise.

A demonstration of this kind can be a rich experience, given that the discussion that follows is thoroughly worked through.

One-way screen demonstrations are technically difficult to conduct: any interaction between teacher and patient or client in the unseen but felt presence of the students is a delicate matter which has to be handled carefully by all parties; and the teaching potential of the method itself is limited by the passive role of the student. The technique can be usefully supplemented by the more active experience of a continuing discussion group, conducted by the same member of the teaching staff over a period of several months, in the course of which personality problems encountered in the clinical material and among the student group can be more fully examined.

It has been objected that much of the foregoing discussion – and, indeed, of discussion in this field generally – is concerned with professional and other competence to deal with *mental illness*, or deviation from the normal; and that little has been said about the imparting of skills that might enhance the individual's capacity for person-to-person relationships. This is a serious shortcoming, because most counselling programmes and psychotherapy in general are concerned with the use of psychological insights to remove blocks in understanding and to minimize personality difficulties, and therefore they operate in the sphere of normality rather than abnormality. Although the training needs of professional people in mental health work whose activities are required only when people are in some kind of difficulty are distinct from the training needs of those whose activities are continuous – such as schoolteachers, whose objectives include that of helping children to grow up as healthy human beings in their own culture – neither group can function adequately without competence in dealing with the normal. The problem here is that the imparting of person-to-person skills within the sphere of normality is handicapped by the comparative lack of knowledge of the psychology of normal people. The views that psychiatrists have of normal people are almost invariably coloured by their experiences with the abnormal.

The Study Group agreed that up to now the essential processes involved in arriving at understanding of dynamic concepts – or what might be termed dynamic understanding – have been explored only very sketchily. In this connexion we hardly know how far it is possible to rely on the mere imparting of intellectual information or on the acquisition by the learner of concepts taken out of their living context. We understand little about the problems that may ensue if the student becomes emotionally involved in the learning process, or even whether adequate learning is possible in the absence of the emotional involvement of the student. We are here on the threshold of the whole problem of the acquisition of insight, a part of learning theory that is still undeveloped – specifically, insight into common human nature in its many different aspects.

The shortage, in most parts of the world, of mental health professional personnel and candidates coming forward for mental health training makes it imperative that training methods should be capable of working effectively with people in their present state of knowledge, in order to make the most economical use of all who are available. We shall be returning to a further discussion of core curricula in Chapter 10. To close this section we note that it is unlikely that students' basic attitudes can be changed by a comparatively brief training programme, but that it is reasonable to expect that their techniques and skills in handling patients can be improved and new ones acquired without, necessarily, extensive modification of their fundamental attitudes. How to increase the number and quality of the people available is a different order of question, and perhaps the most critical task facing us today.

THE TEACHING PROFESSION

Among the professions in which significant advances have been made in mental health training in recent years, perhaps the most notable is the teaching profession. Almost everywhere reports on the training of teachers make reference to one or other aspect of mental health training, although it may be expected that older teachers are no more affected by these new ideas than are their contemporaries in the medical and psychological professions.

The part of UNESCO in fostering mental health aspects of the training and practice of teachers deserves special mention. There are various references in the literature to significant developments in teachers' training colleges, in special educational facilities, school counselling, and so on (439, 442, 619). In a working paper, Morris wrote:

'While as yet only about half the world's children ever attend any kind of school, the proportion coming within organized educational care is everywhere increasing, and the time spent in formal education is everywhere being lengthened. This gives to teachers and others concerned with the conduct of schools and educational systems an increasingly important share of responsibility for the mental health of future generations.

In modern education stress is laid upon personal development through learning. Understanding of children and of the relationships they establish with children in learning situations therefore becomes of paramount concern to teachers. As part of this concern they need to have some appreciation of those practices that are likely to be beneficial to sound development, and of those that may be detrimental to it. It also becomes part of the competence of teachers to be able to recognize signs of maladjustment and difficulty, and to know what resources they may call upon for help. It is therefore of special importance that those responsible for the training of teachers should themselves have an adequate understanding of mental health principles and should be enabled to keep in touch with the developments in the mental health field.'

The Study Group endorsed this statement and drew particular attention to the effect of the learning experience in school on the child's personality development. It underlined the value of the early recognition in schools of signs of maladjustment or difficulty, which will be achieved only if familiarity with mental health principles and their application is an integral part of the teacher's equipment. Although we have remarked on the impossibility of teaching mental health as a curriculum subject, this is not to say that the principles of mental health should not be taught in this way. On the whole teachers, though alive to the concept and value of mental health, are not fully aware, in most parts of the world, of their responsibility for promoting it.

An interesting experiment was reported from Taiwan, where teachers were set to investigate the epidemiology of behavioural disturbances in schools, and at the same time a study was made of the effects on the teachers of their experience and of the instruction in mental health principles that was given concurrently.

The Study Group recommended, for the attention of WFMH, that increased efforts should be made to ensure that those engaged in the training of teachers acquired an adequate understanding of mental health principles and kept in close touch with developments in the mental health field.

The contribution that teachers can make to the mental health of the community goes far beyond the recognition of maladjustment or difficulty in children. The education system of the community can help to establish a sense of values and can promote the emotional and psychological maturation of children. The educational process needs to be in tune both with community values in a wide sense and with the values of the home. It appeared to the Study Group that in many, if not most, parts of the world communication between school, community, and home may not be adequate. A key factor affecting the mental health contribution of the schoolteacher is that of his motivation for entry into the teaching profession.

There is extensive evidence that traditional educational practices are out of touch with current community values and with the emotional needs of children in this modern age. We conclude this chapter with an extended transcript of some notes compiled for the Study Group by Morris, which set out current problems in perspective:

1. Morris draws attention to the very considerable progress that

has been made in a number of countries during the present century, in modifying educational processes and adapting them to modern knowledge of child development and the principles of mental health. But he also points to the immense tasks of reform that are still waiting to be accomplished. There has been an enormous additional complication of programme planning through the rapid quantitative expansion of educational provision throughout the world. Education is changing from being a commodity in short supply, and therefore restricted on class, religious, and 'racial' criteria, to one in potentially abundant supply. Problems of education in relation to mental health are particularly acute in the newly developing countries of Asia, Africa, and Central and South America.

2. The extent to which educational practice still runs counter to mental health requirements in contemporary urban industrial societies may be illustrated by reference to the United Kingdom but, as Morris remarks, some but not all of those features can be found in most other countries.

(i) The curricula and teaching methods are almost exclusively adult-centred, despite great improvements at the school entry stage. The major emphasis is still on 'teaching' rather than on 'learning', and hence on 'instruction' rather than on 'education'.

(ii) Educationists lay more stress on the efficiency of children at their current level than on long-term competence. The widespread use of statistical averages as mandatory norms – as in annual promotion tests – results in a higher value being set on average or class attainments than on the setting of goals for individuals.

(iii) A system of intensive competitive learning over a restricted range of accomplishments (reading, writing, and arithmetic in primary schools, and so-called academic subjects in secondary schools) is resulting in serious deprivation of social, scientific, and aesthetic experience. The majority of children have only minimal experience of cooperative learning, mutual help, and group work.

(iv) Competitive and highly selective examinations, tied to the restricted range referred to above, reinforce the narrowing of experience and lead to anxiety among the children based on adult pressure and expectation. There is a risk that children may suffer the disturbing experience of meeting serious 'failure' at an early age, and as a defence against feared failure may develop unsound attainments based on mechanical skills, memorizing, and highly practised verbal responses without adequate understanding.

(v) The use, almost exclusively, of external (adult-imposed) discipline, as opposed to discipline arising from tasks and mediated by the group, leads to both overdevelopment and underdevelopment of internal controls, and to relative failure to become deeply interested in activities and achievements for their own sake.

(vi) There is a widespread use in schools of systems of control through punishment and correction that are largely unrelated to children's situations and problems, or even to their sense of values, and are related primarily to adult convenience, idiosyncrasy, or anxiety. There may be little or no insight into the role of unconscious adult complicity in producing undesirable behaviour among children.

(vii) A state of continual conflict between pupils (and parents) and the school authority over petty restrictions in school (e.g. dress in adolescence) and over unimportant offences both results from and contributes to failure on the part of the authority to give gradual but continuously increasing responsibility to pupils for school work and organization.

(viii) Failure in school, college, and home to make proper provision for helping adolescents to deal with the conflicts ensuing on the prolongation of social immaturity after arrival at physical sexual maturity is a major cause of adolescent and teenage problems over authority, independence, sexual behaviour, etc.

3. Some of the effects of these practices can be seen in:

(i) The dissatisfaction of many teenagers with their prolonged schooling (in the United Kingdom soon to be prolonged even further) and their lack of abiding interest in what they learnt in school. Their attempts – which, contrary to popular impression, are by no means always ineffective or antisocial – to create their own culture and roles in the social vacuum which they encounter after leaving school form a related yet different and wider issue.

(ii) The relatively large number of mental health 'problems' that are encountered among young people at school, college, and work. We are referring here to problems not as estimated simply by official figures for maladjustment, serious mental illness, or crime, but as known personally to teachers, parents, social workers, and others in touch with the young.

(iii) The relatively immature level of behaviour of large numbers of university and college students, in the intellectual and the emotional spheres.

(iv) The relatively low morale of the teaching profession, which tends to be preoccupied with status, pay, and the search for both internal and external scapegoats. It is relevant to inquire about the relative prevalence of mental ill health among members of the teaching profession.

FURTHER EDUCATION OF
TEACHERS IN MENTAL HEALTH PRINCIPLES

In his working paper Morris remarks that initial training and further education (in-service training) may be considered together, as far as principles are concerned:

1. More effective preparation of teachers for promoting the aims of mental health is not to be thought of simply in terms of increasing their awareness of mental health 'issues' and 'aspects' of their work. Methods of presenting the study of human development are needed, which will enable teachers to deepen their understanding of children, of themselves, and of the nature of the

educational task, in terms which are in harmony with mental health criteria.

2. The ways in which such a preparation can be effectively made depend upon the stage of development which the students have reached themselves, upon the programme of training, the competence and level of maturity of the tutors, and the 'climate' of the training institution.

(i) *The students* are extremely diverse in respect of background and level of maturity, yet they tend to have a common basic attitude to their future job of teaching, which they envisage mainly as a matter of 'putting my subject across and keeping discipline'. These students may be numbered among the successful products of highly intellectualized academic education, and it may be said of them that at entry to training college they are further from understanding childhood – their own and other people's – than they ever have been in the past or will be later. They are almost entirely lacking in sophistication of thought about the biological, psychological, and sociological aspects of human behaviour.

(ii) *The programme:* Developmental studies can occupy only a portion of their time. How can a fruitful beginning best be made? (It can be only a beginning.) Three basic aims are suggested:

(a) To deepen the students' self-awareness and sympathy with others through reflection on their own development, their own anxieties and hopes, their failures and triumphs; through personal observation of children at work and play; through explorations in the recollected world of childhood (autobiographies, etc.); and through acquaintance with the more important facts and major hypotheses of child study and educational psychology.

(b) To foster understanding among the students that education is a process of personal development through achieving mastery of the art and skill of living and learning. The students need to acquire an understanding of school subjects and activities in terms of what the pupils bring to their studies and of what their studies do for pupils.

(c) To develop the insight of students into their role *vis-à-vis* the children (and their own colleagues), and into their own feelings and responses in the teaching situation.

These training aims have to be attempted in the already over-loaded context of practical vocational preparation for work in schools which largely do not yet subscribe to such aims. More-over, it is essential that such studies be intellectually respect-able – that is, they must command the respect of the students who have gone through a highly intellectualized system of academic education. The methods used, on the other hand, must be closely related to the aims proposed, which in many respects relate more closely to feeling tone than to intellect. Before decisions can be made about the scope of formal study methods in these training programmes, there are a number of open and difficult questions to be discussed. For example, to what extent is a fully explicit understanding of psychodynamic concepts required? Can the necessary insights be developed at a less abstract level? How far is unformulated, intuitive understanding sufficient? Whatever the balance of explicit and implicit understanding required, how much can reasonably be expected of an initial training course? (There will be little doubt about the need for later in-service training.) However much is attempted, the effective quality of learning remains the paramount consideration; hence the emphasis on the use of group discussions and of personal tutorials. Clearly education tutors hold a key role.

(iii) *The tutors:* There are a number of questions to be answered about who will be employed: for example, who trains tutors, where do they get experience and what personal qualities do they need to have? Can their role be clearly defined? What principles should guide their work in meeting individual prob-lems, in dealing with students' defences and avoiding the creation of unresolved dependencies, and in steering their tricky educational course between instruction and therapy?

(iv) *The climate of the training institution:* The optimum is hard to define, but, like the school climate it is hoped students will themselves later help to create, it must offer both security and challenge. Individual students vary greatly in the proportions of the admixture of security and challenge that bring out the best in them, and in the best training institutions the individual should be able to find the proportion that he needs, over a wide range. In an optimum atmosphere there must be an insistence on intellectual honesty, and a respect for both corporate and individual values, so that disagreements and tensions between staff and students, and among staff and students respectively, must be acknowledged and worked through. Above all, it is important that the interaction between staff and students should exemplify the essential educational and mental health principles that are taught in the institution.

How this difficult and complicated objective can be attained is a question of primary concern, but by no stretch of the imagination is it within the proper scope of this present volume.

10

Towards a Common Training Policy

After a widely ranging discussion concerning professional roles in and training for mental health work, the Study Group set down a list of seven statements and questions, with the object of delineating some areas for further examination:

1. Professional roles differ widely from area to area and, though they may often have a common label, the effect can be quite misleading.

2. A distinction can properly be drawn between those who are in the focus of mental health work, i.e. who are primarily concerned with it, and those on the periphery, who come into incidental contact with it.

3. It is valuable to distinguish three functions – diagnostic, therapeutic, and follow-up. Should these functions be provided by the same person, or should they be separated?

4. What use can be made of existing local facilities in training programmes in 'psychiatrically underdeveloped' areas? What use should be made of expatriate training, and at which stages in the process?

5. Where there are several professional groups involved, to what extent is it possible to provide for common training in some respects? That is, how far is it feasible to develop a core curriculum, and over what range should a core curriculum extend?

6. In programmes of professional training at the focus of mental health work, what are the best techniques to deal with problems arising in the early days of training from the personal

emotional involvement of students in what they are learning and in the patient–therapist relationship? What proportions of such training should be in an academic and in a practical setting respectively?

7. What can be done at a transnational level about virtually universal reports of shortages of professional personnel and the need to improve the quality of trainees?

The idea of providing more training in common for the professions both at the focus and at the periphery of mental health work has a considerable appeal, because it appears to promise economy of effort as well as a widening of the individual student's horizon. There are drawbacks, however: a potential disadvantage of the communal training experience is that what the student gains in the widening of his experience and sympathy may be offset by a lowering of the standard he reaches in a particular subject. Medical teachers in a number of countries are familiar with this difficulty, from the common practice of combining the training of students of anatomy, physiology, and pharmacology with that of medical students in these subjects, to the detriment of all parties. The science students tend to be kept at a lower technical level in these subjects than they would otherwise attain, and the medical students tend to be overloaded with material that is not relevant to their later clinical needs, and may be presented to them in a way that is unrelated to the use to which they will put their knowledge later on, by teachers not fully in sympathy with the ultimate objectives of the training.

The extent to which the diverse interests of the students can be turned to advantage in the more didactic aspects of teaching is limited, particularly in the early training in those basic sciences that are common to the various professional disciplines. The teaching of combined groups of students of different orientations has often proved unsatisfactory, partly because of the compromises that have to be made and partly because the areas of common usage of basic sciences may be less than is often supposed.

The Study Group, attempting to arrive at some principles that might govern the effectiveness of programmes of training in common, suggested that the most valuable advantage of shared training by students of various professions might lie in the variety of previous experience that the students bring with them, which can enrich the learning processes of the whole group. It is generally the case that students of the basic sciences and pre-clinical medical students have little variety to offer to each other in terms of their past experience. Thus, one of the most useful mutual learning techniques – that of role-playing – is inapplicable at this stage of training because there is insufficient diversity of previous role experience among the students.

In the more academic aspects of professional training as opposed to basic science training it has also proved difficult to combine the needs of two or more student groups. For example, it is common practice to admit social worker students to medical students' lectures on social medicine, or medical students to certain parts of psychology courses. But unless there is a great deal of adaptation to the visitors' needs, which may not be possible without disadvantage to the host group, such practices are of little value, in our opinion. They may even be harmful should they raise misconceptions, and later prejudices, in the students' minds about other disciplines.

On the other hand, there have been many examples of the successful mixing of disciplines in the more clinical aspects of training. The central concern here is not so much the assumed existence of a common field of study for members of different professions as the provision of a meeting ground to which the professions can each bring their own specific experience to the discussion of problems in common. Clinical demonstrations and seminar discussions attended by members of various professional disciplines are capable of providing a training experience that has a different meaning for each class of participant. Each category of student has a specific role or part to play. Each brings to the common discussion the particular contribution of his own experience and each has an opportunity to learn about the experience, attitudes, and needs of the other students.

There is no general agreement about what is the best time during training for mental health work to introduce elements in common to two or more categories of student. In many countries it is usual to separate the so-called basic sciences from the more clinical or practical aspects of training, and to require that the student first pass through the basic courses more or less without reference to what is to follow. Education practices vary widely from country to country in these respects, the variations no doubt being related to what goes on in the schools. Where, as in many countries, school education is solely and exclusively didactic in conception and presentation, it is hardly likely that universities will be responsive to suggestions that other methods might be introduced into the teaching of the basic sciences. On the other hand, universities may well be receptive to innovations in the case of clinical subjects, which obviously demand a style of presentation different from that of traditional didactic teaching.

Many educationists advocate the introduction of learner participation and common training sessions through the medium of role-playing in case discussions during the final year at school, in preparation for university. There are interesting experiments in which pupils studying the sciences, the humanities, modern languages, and classics get together for a common discussion of a practical subject – for example, 'citizenship' – and each pupil is given the opportunity to contribute his own specific attitude. Where such sophisticated attitudes are prevalent in schools, the universities are likely to follow, as the new generation of students begins to take up teaching posts in the universities. (Mental health teaching in schools is discussed more fully in a later section.)

The Study Group was of the opinion that common training experiences in mental health principles and practice are valuable for medical students, medical auxiliaries, nurses, psychologists, dentists, and pharmacists. The last-named are important, though they are usually overlooked in this connexion, because it is so often the retail pharmacist who forms the first line of defence against the individual's real, feared, or imagined illness. A very great number of people will consult the pharmacist first about some symptom, or will answer an advertisement in a newspaper. The Study Group also thought that common learning experiences could be widely applied in the social and educational services.

CORE CURRICULUM

In addition to the provision of training experiences in common at the practical or clinical level, we have referred briefly above to more basic and formal common training programmes for students of professions both at the focus and at the periphery of mental health work. We should like to discuss further some of the possibilities of core curricula – those aspects of training that can be equally relevant to all the professions concerned, and might be organized into formal courses of study. This idea when first encountered is very attractive, but, as in the case of less formal training practices, the technical difficulties are considerable. Obviously, the more homogeneous the objectives of the professions, the more relevant the core curriculum, and it is logical to suggest that though the possibility may be worth further exploration in the case of the professions at the focus of mental health work, it is hardly likely to be useful in the case of those at the periphery.

Among the subjects put forward as relevant to a core curriculum for professions primarily concerned with mental health are: human biology, genetics, some aspects of comparative animal biology, developmental psychology, sociology, some aspects of social anthropology, bio-statistics, and psychopathology. Among the subjects of a more clinical or applied type that are shared by these professions are: human relations (individual and group), human personality studies, casework principles, and the dynamics of the interview.

The Study Group was inclined to the view that attempts to establish more formal core curricula would encounter difficulties similar to, if not greater than, those noted in respect of less highly organized common training experiences. That is, the varying needs of the different professional disciplines for the elaboration of basic subjects and their special interests in particular subjects might prove to a large extent incompatible. We have already referred to the danger of confusing the standards expected of the various categories of student, when two or more professions are being taught together.

A core curriculum in respect of the basic sciences would appear to be most applicable in the early stages of the course, when students are less likely to bring widely varying levels of sophistication to the study. Systems of this kind are in use at the present time in a number of universities for the teaching of the human sciences, but it is probably fair to remark that they have been introduced rather as a means of economizing on the time and energy of the teaching staff than as a deliberate measure in the design of the individual student's course.

Not least of the difficulties in the way of international discussion of this subject is the enormous variation to be found, in different countries, in university courses purporting to have the same objective. Some illustrations can be given: in Australia, it is possible to enter immediately, as an undergraduate, a three-year training in clinical psychology; whereas in South Africa the individual must obtain an arts or a science degree before he can proceed to a special professional training in clinical, personnel, or educational psychology. In the United Kingdom the practice is more akin to the South African than the Australian, but there is no uniformity. In the United States, probably to a greater extent than in other countries, there is in most professions a tendency to require a general arts or science degree before the student can proceed to a further degree in his special subject. This is so in the case of medical training in the United States and, whereas in the United Kingdom requirements vary according to the university, it is possible in a number of medical schools for medical students to receive training only in strictly medical subjects (the preclinical studies being narrowly technological). Another variation in university practice which is found in some countries of continental Europe is that of spending successive periods in different universities while studying for a particular degree. Still another example of disparity of practice is the extent to which some of the professions are being trained outside university circles altogether. This applies particularly to social work and nursing. In some countries university degrees are unknown in either of these subjects, in some they are facultative and reserved for an élite, and in others they are more or less obligatory for all.

The ramifications of modern medicine are so wide that it may be more objective to regard medicine as a complex of distinctive professions whose training is everywhere based on a core curriculum; yet when one considers how distinctive the various medical specialities are – the width of the range of activities into which medical graduates divide themselves after qualification – the conclusion appears inescapable that no single medical speciality is served by the type of training that is best suited to it. At least this will be generally accepted in the case of the clinical specialities, ranging from general practice through specialized surgery and internal medicine to obstetrics, gynaecology, paediatrics, psychosomatic medicine, general psychiatry, and child psychiatry.

Many of the difficulties hindering the introduction of mental health principles into medical training today are of historical origin, and for this reason are perhaps all the more resistant to rational change. The fact is that physical, biochemical, and pharmacological techniques have become much more highly developed than psychological techniques, and it is very difficult for a profession that is supported by a number of highly advanced sciences to be open to influences coming from a science that appears to be less developed.

Whatever the difficulties, it is clear that some forms of core curricula in the basic studies of the various professions are already in existence in many countries, and, moreover, for many reasons, they are likely to spread. The whole field deserves further study.

There are certain subjects which, although they are of only limited interest as far as particular trainees are concerned, are essential because of their contribution to the understanding of the main field of knowledge. These might be regarded – metaphorically – as the vitamins of professional training. An example of this type of subject is statistics, for it is probably the case that one cannot advance far in general psychology or sociology, or in medicine in its public health, biochemical, and therapeutic aspects, without being able to handle statistical data in at least an elementary way. Another example is psychopathology, for although knowledge of this subject, like that of statistics, is required by the different professions at very different levels of complexity, comparatively little can be learnt about mental health without a grasp of the elementary concepts of psychopathology, human dynamism, and environmental factors, and little practical success will be gained without some competence in dealing with psychological dysfunction.

We might add another metaphorical vitamin which, like many more concrete biochemical substances, cannot be isolated as yet, but its presence can be inferred from observation of its effects. This analogy should not be taken too far – but in the course of professional education it may be observed that nearly all students will develop an individuality that is different from that of their starting-point. Such development can best be achieved when the individual is sufficiently free from rigidities and dependency to be able to draw fully on his own potential, or, in the words of a psychologist in the Group, on his humanity. The training influences and experiences that are necessary in this connexion are those that serve to augment the humanity of the student, in order not so much that he may function better, but that he may function *at all*, in this field. In other words, this is a matter of personality growth and development whereby the individual attains insight and understanding. What is meant here by insight and understanding may be illustrated in a negative way by citing the example of those many people who know a great deal about children, but who never demonstrate that they are capable of understanding one single living child. It can hardly be supposed that this unisolable vitamin can be prescribed as an ingredient of any core curriculum. But, if the analogy will stand being taken one step further, it is not unreasonable to seek to supply it empirically in the general nutriment of the student, which it may not be possible to do successfully without the aid of a suitable atmosphere in school education.

In Chapter 14 (p. 262) we shall return to the discussion of the function of schools in preparing students for professional work in these fields, but it is relevant to note here that more use could be made of the traditional educational source of literature for the imparting of insights and the development of awareness. This, it is emphasized, is a very different matter from the study of psychopathology through literature as a curriculum subject; it is rather the direction of the student's mind towards the possibility of understanding motivation and feeling through the insights of the author.

Another aspect of professional training to which greater attention should be paid concerns the tendency common to students of a number of the professions involved to enter a phase of distrust of their spontaneous reactions to circumstances, without having yet assimilated into their thinking the scientific or technical principles that they are studying. Many students dare not trust their own judgement and they seek rules they can slavishly apply, in which mood they are apt to be blinded by the appearance of science. Unfortunately, a minority never fully emerge from this phase, and thus they add to the ranks of those who fail to reach a full understanding, though their knowledge may be profound. It appears to us that this is an aspect of training to which the clinical demonstration in common, to which students bring their own insights, can make a key contribution.

Even a brief examination reveals the enormous complexities of curriculum-building for mental health education. The more one surveys the field, the more one is likely to be appalled by what the student is required to do. The situation calls for a careful scrutiny to determine, on the one hand, how much it is reasonable to expect students to have assimilated by the end of the training period and, on the other, how much it is realistic to attempt to teach them in the limited time available. This is a current educational dilemma. The Study Group agreed that no kind of professional training presumes to turn out a professional person fully equipped in all respects at the end of the training period, and that training plans should be constructed with this limitation clearly in mind. This means that the educational process cannot reach a finality of definition in terms of content. Concern with content is not enough; in this field it is imperative to think more about educational principles and processes.

The conclusion of the Study Group about the introduction of the so-called core curriculum was that its greatest potential value lay in the improvement it could be expected to bring with respect to communications between the various professions. The processes of devising and introducing curricula are, admittedly, of great complexity and must vary according to professional needs and university practices in different countries. Many points strike the mental health sophisticate with a glaring obviousness – e.g. the inadequate teaching of psychology in medical schools almost all over the world; the absence of human relations concepts in teaching. Each profession could probably make for itself a list of pressing needs, and it is clear that all the professions concerned have much to do to set their own houses in order.

Nevertheless, we must discover more about the basic requirements for working in the field of mental health, and learn how to increase the common background and to improve the means of communication between people of different professional disciplines. The Study Group recommended strongly to the World Federation for Mental Health that further studies should be sponsored to determine the basic material from various fields – including psychology, sociology, biology, etc. – that should go into the training of people working in the sciences of man.

COMMUNITY LEADERS

In the period since 1948 there has been a patchy development of programmes for the mental health education of professional and semi-professional people occupying positions of influence in the social relations of the community, but not directly involved in mental health work. In some parts of the world this trend has reached quite significant proportions, but in most areas it is hardly apparent. In addition to general practitioners, public health personnel, and teachers – who have already been mentioned in this connexion – ministers of religion, staffs of institutions, police, welfare workers, some court officials, e.g. probation officers, and, in some instances, lawyers, have been in receipt of training in mental health principles.

A remarkable pioneer effort has been made in the State of Victoria, Australia, in devising systematic programmes with the object of orientating community leaders to the mental health problems inherent in their own work. It is hoped there to create in the current generation an informed public opinion, which may become the common property of the next generation. Where, as in Victoria, such a programme has been coupled with consultant services to general practitioners, educational services, a large group of social welfare agencies, children's and adult courts, well-baby clinics, and so on, the result has been a marked improvement in the attitudes of professional people towards the problems of mental health. This has led to a community reorientation regarding questions of the early detection and management of mental ill health, and it has enabled the development of a more positive mental health programme based on the community's own values.

The Study Group discussed the special needs of ministers of religion in relation to the use that might be made of mental health principles. A clergyman member of the Group urged a more concerted effort to make available to religious groups relevant new information from medicine, social sciences, and other behavioural sciences. A wide field of relevance can be envisaged. For example, modern medical techniques are tending to place the whole question of deterioration and death in a different light, and preoccupation with health and eradication of disease may affect people's attitudes to death and dying in a very marked way. In a society in which old people are living longer, the need for greater understanding of the dynamics of human relations might become more acute. The new corpus of knowledge that is being developed in the field of mental health is potentially of the greatest relevance to the work of the minister of religion, and considerable advantages might accrue from application of this knowledge, not only by religious educators, but also by the members of several other professions, notably lawyers. Although members of the legal professions, and particularly judges and advocates, are notoriously resistant to concepts of mental health, especially when dynamic psychological principles are involved, many are now realizing for themselves the potential injustice and inhumanity of attempting to handle divorce cases and problems of the custody of children by a rigid application of precedents determined by the so-called legal rights of the parents. They are finding that, on the contrary, their work takes them right into the middle of emotional and even psychiatric problems.

As Ewalt pointed out in a working paper, referring primarily to the United States:

'Studies of manpower available now and in the foreseeable future clearly show that physicians, nurses, social workers, and psychologists are now in short supply, and will be increasingly so in the next several years. The United States population is growing rapidly and the numbers and kinds of persons and agencies wanting psychiatric facilities are increasing. These two factors at work in the health profession apply equally to the sciences, to teaching, the law, and the clergy.'

There are many countries similarly placed, and the need to ensure that all persons who are professionally dealing with people should have a sound grounding in mental health principles is being progressively recognized. The Study Group agreed that, since the work of all these professional groups – physicians, lawyers, teachers, religious leaders, nurses, social workers, and community leaders – has implications for mental health, all those engaged in professional training in these areas should be encouraged to give increased attention to the fields of psychiatry and the social sciences, so that the contribution of these fields to the improvement of professional practice can be secured for the benefit of the community.

MENTAL HEALTH AND DIPLOMACY

The question has been raised in recent years as to how mental health insights and skills can be effectively applied to the field of diplomacy, particularly in the sphere of international relations. In general, it is valid to state that the conduct of diplomats has been formalized by several centuries of practical experience, and it is based on a more or less rigid code which has something of the function of an international language, or at least a standardized means of communication.

On the whole, diplomats tend, conventionally, to regard differences that they may become aware of as deriving from culture rather than from individual personality; in other words, to apply national stereotypes. It has sometimes happened that when a diplomat with an idiosyncratic or deviant personality has occupied a key position in international relations, a great deal of difficulty has ensued. It may well be a fact that disastrous wars have occurred because of personality factors in leading individuals that have remained unrecognized or have been misinterpreted by diplomats.

These are complex issues. It is obviously impracticable to propose that behavioural scientists be given a place, as of professional right, in international channels of negotiation. Not only would such a proposal cut across centuries of usage and thus stand little or no chance of success, but the proposal itself could not be justified objectively except in circumstances when the behavioural scientists themselves were of proven competence in the field in which they would have to operate. The fact that present diplomats are not, with very rare exceptions, professionally competent in the understanding of human motivation and the science of communication, does not itself validate the intervention of the behavioural scientist.

The Study Group thought that the most fruitful mental

health contribution in this area would be to help the diplomats concerned to gain better insights into human personality and behaviour, and to understand more about the sociodynamics of international communication. In this connexion attention is drawn to a series of residential seminars for diplomats of various nationalities, organized during recent years, on behalf of the American Society of Friends, at Clarens, Switzerland. These seminars have been designed for younger diplomats who appear to be likely to achieve high office later, and have been attended by invitation. Programmes have ranged freely within the general topic of 'The Role of Diplomacy in a Changing World'. There have been three main streams of discussion – the economic, the political, and the psychological aspects of the diplomat's job.

Though the quantitative effect of such seminars may be quite small, their potential effect is incalculable. One of the most encouraging results has been the establishment of a chain of communication between a number of individuals in the various foreign services and diplomatic missions who have had personal experience, as members of a transcultural group, of exploring these matters of interpersonal relationships.

There have been a number of other attempts on a small scale to interest younger people working in the diplomatic field in the question of personality variations and, in particular, in the possibility of personality changes due to emotional disturbances or developing disorders. A third approach, described in Volume I and referred to in the Introductory to this volume, has been the attempt by the World Federation for Mental Health, with the collaboration of the Carnegie Foundation among other organizations, to impart mental health insights to members of national delegations to the United Nations and the UN specialized agencies, through the convening of meetings and discussion groups. On occasion an expert in the field of the behavioural sciences has been included in a country's mission, more with the role of interpreting behaviour to the other members of the team than as a participant in the determination of policy.

Such efforts to bring mental health insights into the field of diplomacy are having a reserved reception, on the whole. The notion of including mental health experts in missions traditionally regarded as the preserve of people with quite other types of experience naturally evokes a defensive reaction. Moreover, it cannot be denied that at present the introduction of considerations of human dynamics into diplomatic discussions complicates rather than expedites decisions, because it brings into the area of discussion a whole range of additional factors with which the diplomatic team is unfamiliar.

The Study Group agreed that the difficulties inherent in a direct application of mental health principles to diplomatic procedures are such that a more indirect approach is to be preferred – mainly through improved selection methods and the education of diplomats in these matters. In a number of countries a start has been made with the employment of more scientific techniques for the selection of the more responsible cadres of diplomatic officials. Selection procedures are concerned with two aspects: the detection and elimination of personality types considered to be unsuitable, and the prediction of qualities of leadership and ability to take responsibility among the candidates.

In addition to studying selection procedures, Torre has described in a working paper the training of personnel in government service in interpersonal relations by the use of group discussion sessions to which the psychiatrist contributes his professional insight. Torre points out that understanding of variations in normal behaviour is most useful in such tasks as getting people to cooperate in technical assistance projects and to participate in conferences.

Torre has developed for officials a technique of group discussions to deal with problems caused by those common medical and psychiatric conditions that tend to alter personality and behaviour. He remarks that it is usually not difficult to get agreement to the proposition that success in interpersonal understanding depends upon each party fulfilling more or less what the other parties expect of him; and that personality disturbance and emotional disorders may so transform the patterns of behaviour that serious misunderstandings arise which might be avoided if there were more awareness among the participants.

Torre has found these methods to be helpful to officials in the recognition of such conditions as depression and pathological anxiety, and also of those changes in personality that accompany the medical conditions common in middle age and chronic diseases. He points out that, without in any sense being turned into psychiatrists, diplomats can be helped to acquire much more skill in recognizing the presence of irrational behaviour and in knowing how to deal with it in the work situation.

II
The Special Needs of Developing Areas

THE PSYCHIATRICALLY DEVELOPING COUNTRIES

Much of the discussion about training so far has referred implicitly to societies where there is a high standard of general medical education, a tradition of psychiatric specialization, and a reasonably effective level of organization of social welfare services. It is timely now to consider some of the special training problems that exist in countries where mental health action is in a far less developed state. Even the limited amount of experience that has been gained so far has made it very clear that countries that are newly emerging in these regards require quite specific programmes, designed for their particular situation, for the training of professional personnel and for the more general educational preparation of the public in these matters.

It is generally agreed that it is largely inappropriate – or even futile – for countries where mental health services are rudimentary or just beginning to recapitulate all the developmental stages of countries where such services have been longer established. An illustration can be taken from the comparatively long tradition of mental welfare work in the United Kingdom. Here, acceptance by the community of responsibility for the provision of public hospitals for the mentally ill, which has grown from small initiatives about 150 years ago, is itself based on an earlier tradition, dating back some 400 years to the so-called Poor Law legislation, which acknowledged community responsibility for citizens in need. So that preventive mental health services in the United Kingdom, which have slowly and somewhat tortuously emerged, via a proliferation of large mental hospitals more or less remote from the community they serve, to embrace all the modern paraphernalia of preventive mental health action in the community, are also grounded in tradition nearly four centuries old. In another country, in which there has been no tradition of community care for the needy, it would be inadvisable to attempt to follow a similar pattern – that is, to set up large hospital buildings – on the way towards the establishment of preventive services. Yet this is precisely what is tending to happen in developing countries, as legislators, becoming aware of the problem of mental disorder in their midst, are tempted to copy what appear to them to be the most useful aspects of other countries' mental health services. This point was made very clear in an illuminating contribution to the WHO seminar on mental health in Africa, held in Brazzaville in 1958 (91).

The existence, in a country, of a well-established professional cadre, including medical personnel, nurses, and social workers, can make a vast difference to the whole course of progress in mental health action in that country. In the absence of one or all of these classes of professional worker, plans for the introduction of mental health work have to be specifically devised in order to suit the more limited capacity of the community for which they are intended.

An example of recent special planning is provided by events that followed the acquisition of independence by the Congolese Republic, where it was found that there was a very grave shortage of medical personnel. WHO arranged for some seventy health assistants, who had already received three years' training in simple medical care in the Congo, to be given three years' supplementary training in France in order to become qualified medical practitioners. Fortunately, it was arranged that some training in psychiatry and in principles of mental health should be included in this supplementary scheme, with the object of promoting insight in these areas among the practitioners. This programme, though modest in comparison with what is needed for comprehensive psychiatric training, may very possibly add immeasurably to the quality of the work of these key personnel.

TRAINING OF MENTAL HEALTH PERSONNEL
FOR NEW AREAS OF WORK

The training of personnel to work in areas where there has been
no mental health work previously, or only rudimentary activity,
is a complex undertaking that is affected by many variables
deriving from differences in the culture, language, and structure
of the societies involved. Some of the professions engaged in
modern mental health work may have been previously unknown
in the country concerned. One of the first questions to ask is
whether the existing distinctions among professional roles in the
more developed countries, which may have served as a model for
the new undertaking, are relevant to the needs of a country in
which mental health activity is only beginning.

Mead drew attention in a working paper to the many unsolved
problems in the training of mental health personnel for new areas
of work, one of the most difficult being the level at which explicit
psychiatric training should be introduced. Another obstacle to
the promotion of satisfactory training schemes is the geographical
and economic pressures to form regional groups for the training
of personnel, under the general heading of 'South-east Asia' or
'The Caribbean', for example. It is evident that these and other
designated regions do have many relevant features in common;
nevertheless, such generalizations tend to obscure finer differences in family structure, in ethos, in view of the world, all of
which may be very significant in respect of mental health. Mead
further noted the possibility that the preservation of a careful
and explicit respect for differences in cultures may have the
paradoxical effect of giving rise to the formation of generalized
stereotypes, about 'East' and 'West', for example, and about
'nuclear' and 'extended' families in South-east Asia or the 'unstable' family structure of the Caribbean, and so on. These
stereotypes may be advantageous to the extent that they help to
clarify thought and perception, but their undiscriminating
adoption could be inimical to understanding, especially when,
as in the case of generalizations about 'unstable' families, they may
be no more than projections of Western, urban, industrialized,

or middle-class cultural attitudes. Conversely, the new stereotypes depicting the kinds of family that 'go with' urbanization may be adopted by members of new nations moving towards the position of modern industrialized societies, and in this way great and unnecessary violence may be done to existing systems.

The view was strongly supported in the Study Group that mental health education as a preparation for mental health practice in psychiatrically developing countries is the central mental health task of the next decade.

It is difficult to make further generalizations in this connexion, because each country has a unique history and quite specific needs. Hardly any country is completely undeveloped in this area, but in many the provisions are traditional only and hardly recognizable in a modern mental health context. There are wide variations between countries with regard to the length of time their medical schools have been in existence, the level of their public health measures, the extent of their community health services; and also in many other more technical respects, such as their degree of familiarity with and acceptance of psychodynamic thinking.

It is likely that every country that tackles these questions will establish a different order of priorities at the outset. Where there has been a comparatively strong medical tradition, but a weak or non-existent social work tradition, early priority will almost certainly be given to the development of psychiatry and the training of psychiatrists; where an educational emphasis has been stronger, psychology may be accorded some priority. In the great majority of countries, however, the initial preoccupation will be with the more medical aspects. We shall therefore consider these training problems primarily in relation to psychiatry, but much of the discussion is pertinent to all the professions engaged in mental health work.

OVERSEAS TRAINING PROGRAMMES IN PSYCHIATRY

The Study Group expressed concern at the widely prevalent modern practice whereby young medical graduates are sent from their own newly developing countries to other countries for prolonged periods of specialized psychiatric training. This practice has been fostered in recent years by the fellowship training programmes of the United Nations and other agencies; these schemes use universities in many parts of the world and have enabled large numbers of young promising medical personnel, both men and women, to get psychiatric training away from their home countries. These overseas fellowship training schemes are generally defended on two grounds: first, that adequate training facilities are not available in the home country; second, that it is comparatively inexpensive to introduce a few additional students into well-established university centres. It is argued that so long as the trainee has a good grasp of the language of the host country, a proved capacity to adapt to a new cultural environment, and sound psychological defences against anxiety, exile, and loneliness, he has nothing to fear from the experience and a great deal to gain.

Quite apart from the difficulties involved in selecting trainees of such calibre, it is being increasingly realized that an overwhelming disadvantage of training practices of this kind is that there can be no guarantee that the knowledge of psychiatry that the student acquires will be properly relevant to the country of his origin, to which it is the intention that he shall return. The trainee himself will rarely be in a position to realize the essentially exotic nature of much of his new knowledge, nor in most cases will he have the insight and skill required to make the necessary mental adjustment for himself. There is a further danger, of which there have been many instances in recent years, that the overseas trainee, finding himself more and more out of touch with his own culture, but feeling himself technically competent to work in the host country, may be drawn to remain there. The Study Group took the view that, in principle, before going abroad for training, a young psychiatrist should already have arrived at a good understanding of the psychiatric and social problems of his own community, particularly in regard to medical ecology. He should also have spent a considerable time in gaining experience of clinical problems, a period of five years being suggested. In other words, before a psychiatrist goes abroad for training he should have gained adequate insight into the nature of his own best role in psychiatry.

In present circumstances these recommendations may constitute a counsel of unattainable perfection; nevertheless, the point is emphasized that the better the nucleus of psychiatric training at home, the greater the benefit that is likely to be reaped from overseas training experience. In our view, an integral part of any overseas training scheme should be the simultaneous establishment in university settings in the home country of systematically organized training programmes for students of psychiatry and other professions concerned with mental health. It is not enough to attempt to get along, as so often happens today, with in-service training experience gained more or less haphazardly. The question of how local centres can be set up is both complex and urgent. The idea of establishing postgraduate schools of psychiatry may appear hopelessly ambitious in some countries, in the light of their university systems and resources. In such cases there is much to be said for regional training centres, for example, for the Arab-speaking world, or for certain parts of Africa which have a language and some cultural aspects in common, or for South and Central America respectively.

The problem of how to get psychiatric personnel trained in a country where there are very few trained professional workers can hardly be solved by a simple recommendation that psychiatric training should, in principle, be undertaken in the student's own country, and that overseas training should be reserved for later stages of his career. One approach that is often put forward as a means of alleviating the situation entails the reverse procedure – that of importing experienced teachers from another country into the local training centre. Many attempts to put this method into practice have shown, however, the essential difficulties of the undertaking. In addition to the fact that the imported teacher is likely to find the vernacular language a problem, he is almost bound to experience stress in attempting to understand the unfamiliar local culture and in having to compensate for the disadvantage inherent in the foreign image he presents to his students. Another point that must be considered is the motivation of teachers who are prepared to work on short-term agreements in undeveloped areas; there may be complications, too, when they return to their own countries in due course. It may be very difficult to get the receiving country to make adequate arrangements for the foreign teachers. For example, it must be prepared to offer high enough salaries to attract personnel accustomed to a higher standard of living, though such rates of pay will often seem huge in the eyes of the local people. Furthermore, adjustments to housing and living standards may be necessary for the health and efficiency of the visitors, but they also constitute an impediment to the teachers' understanding of the local cultural situation and to the acceptability of the teachers among the local inhabitants.

It has sometimes happened that a country realizes quite suddenly its need for more psychiatric and other mental health training, following disclosures about the amount of mental illness among its people or the poor treatment conditions, or as a result of a growing awareness of how these matters are managed in other countries. Thus there may be a political clamour for immediate action, and the opportunity to send a small cadre of promising young men and women abroad may be eagerly seized upon without proper reflection. Popular pressure may make it impossible to plan on a five- or ten-year basis, although all the indications are that a period of this order is necessary for success. Moreover, it may be difficult, if not impossible, to find agencies in other countries which would be willing to guarantee support for a long-term scheme. Few individuals or agencies are willing to think in terms of five- or ten-year programmes, and very few individuals indeed can contemplate a lifetime in overseas service. In fact, the career problems inherent in long-term schemes may well be insoluble, unless the developing country is able to create confidence that it is prepared to offer lifelong employment to expatriates who are willing to identify with it.

The Study Group advocated the consideration in principle of a two-point plan for introducing higher psychiatric training to a country where these facilities are inadequate or do not exist. The first step is to set up a postgraduate psychiatric training centre in an established medical school. Where no suitable medical school is available, it may be an unavoidable preliminary task to provide one, even at the expense of delaying the psychiatric training by as much as ten years.

The second point is that it can be a tremendous advantage if an appropriate, well-established university in another country where psychiatric training is highly developed is associated with the training plan from the outset. There have been many successful experiences of an older university becoming the sponsor of a newly emerging university in another country, and maintaining with it, for a period of years, a special reciprocal relationship.

The sponsoring university would be responsible, in agreement with the new university, for the recruitment of experienced teachers to form the nucleus of the faculty of the new university. The teachers would, preferably, be recruited from a number of countries, and they would be offered appointments endowed with the prestige of the sponsoring university, which would greatly facilitate secondment; alternatively, they would be guaranteed an academic appointment in their own country upon completion of their term of service.

In the case of most members of the founding teaching staff, the term of service would be for not less than five years in the first instance. This would be a necessary condition, particularly where there was a new language to learn – vernacular communication is an essential in mental health work – and where cultural differences were significant. Only a very limited teaching programme would be practicable during the first year, which the expatriate teaching personnel would devote to language study, cultural orientation, and administrative organization, and to cooperation in the selection of local personnel suitable to be members of a training cadre to be sent overseas. These would be the most promising of the younger men and women, ready for specialization in their professions. They would be selected with a view to undertaking future teaching responsibility so that, on their return, they would, in time, replace the original foreign founding staff. They would go for a period of about two years to training vacancies arranged for them under the general supervision of the sponsoring university, preferably in a number of different countries. At the same time, any postgraduate students belonging to the country who were already abroad would be contacted and offered the opportunity of coordinating their training programmes with a view to their eventual return to join the staff of the new training school. It is possible that, as the training institution grew, it would be useful to retain the services of those expatriate teachers who wished to continue to be associated with it, in order to meet the needs of expanding departments. After the first four years or so, it would no longer be desirable to send personnel overseas for training at an early stage of specialization. During the time that the first cadre was abroad, the founding teaching staff would organize the institution's own training programme so that it could go into full operation when the overseas trainees returned. Subsequently, training overseas would, in principle, be reserved for the acquiring of special types of experience not available locally, and for broadening the conceptual framework of senior postgraduate students.

The successful operation of a training scheme of this order would require a great deal of adaptability both on the part of the foreign staff, who would have to be willing to be diverted from their university careers at home for an indefinite period, and on the part of the students of the country concerned, who would encounter unfamiliar cultural patterns. It is essential for the effectiveness of any such scheme that the sponsoring university should ensure that these expatriate appointments fit into the recognized career structure of the receiving country, and that there is a minimum of anxiety among the recruited staff about their redeployment into university careers at the end of the overseas period. If attention is not given to this last point, the training scheme will tend to recruit only people who have little expectation of securing key appointments in the academic life of their own country.

Little work has been done on the question of preparing trainees for periods of study in foreign countries, although university experience everywhere is that the comparative failure of foreign postgraduate students – to the extent that they fail to reap full benefit from their courses of study – may reach disquietingly large dimensions. The trainee going abroad should be given much more assistance: he needs to be briefed on the conditions he will find in the new country; appropriate arrangements should be made for the continuation of his family life; questions of accommodation and subsistence should be settled in advance; he must feel secure in respect of his long-term career. In addition, there is an increasing realization of the need for what has been termed 'de-briefing', to assist the returning student to reorient himself, so that he will be able to apply what he has learnt to the conditions of his own country to the best advantage, and not merely carry over, unchanged, the foreign attitudes he has acquired. It is not an exaggeration to remark that the process of de-briefing should, ideally, be put in train before the student leaves his own country on the outward journey. The first step is to ensure that the departing student is not entirely unsophisticated about cultural differences. The teachers in the foreign country must themselves be aware of the issues involved, and it is highly desirable that someone who has an intimate knowledge of conditions in the student's home culture should be freely accessible to him for consultation during his residence abroad. Because the training experience will provide an immense amount of material in the cultural sphere to be worked through, the process of de-briefing needs to be continued for some months, if not years, after the student's return to his own country; consultation, group discussion, and other techniques may be employed for this purpose.

We have outlined one way of establishing a psychiatric training centre where none has previously existed. Many other kinds of 'bilateral' arrangements might be made between two countries with different resources, strengths, and weaknesses, with the objective of forming an ongoing association for the exchange of professional personnel and training to their mutual advantage.

THE ROLE OF THE VISITING FOREIGN EXPERT

Just as the value of sending students abroad at an early stage of their professional education is now seriously questioned, so the concept of the visiting foreign 'expert' or consultant is being subjected to critical examination. There appears to be mounting dissatisfaction with the practice of commissioning a foreign expert to make a short visit to a country, report on its needs, and make recommendations. It has been suggested that the primary, and perhaps the only really valid, functions of the visiting expert are to stimulate the people in the less developed country to think and act for themselves, and to support and give added prestige to the work of local pioneers. Many of the negative criticisms that are made about consultant visits are due, the Group considered, to the fact that criteria for the selection of consultants are lacking, and to the joint failure of the promoters and the consultants to conceptualize what is really wanted and to formulate precise plans.

In general, the conditions that have to be met before foreign consultants can be successful are inadequately understood and catered for. For example, although it is acknowledged that those who go abroad on missions for periods of less than two years do not undertake the learning of an unfamiliar language, very little consideration is given to what level of mental health work can reasonably be undertaken without a knowledge of the local language. In the case of short-term missions the choice of consultant may have to be restricted to people who already know the language, which is a prohibitive condition in most instances. A very poor alternative is to rely on the services of an interpreter: the resulting communication cannot be compared with the process of consultation achieved by the expert working in the vernacular. It is probably useful for a distinguished visitor to bring his experience to bear on the broad problems of a particular country, but the quality of his understanding may be seriously impaired if he is unable to appreciate the emotional subtleties of communication.

There are frequent complaints to the effect that a country has not made adequate preparations for the reception of a foreign expert; indeed, there may be no general agreement about how he is to be treated. In some instances there may be a political contest to gain proprietary rights over the consultant; in other cases he may be kept at arm's length by everyone and regarded as an individual apart; he may even be placed in a virtual ghetto if it is usual for his fellow nationals to be somewhat isolated in that country. Often there is a lack of precision regarding the lines of communication that are available to the visiting consultant, his access to the appropriate government official, and the arrangements for acting upon his recommendations.

NON-MEDICAL MENTAL HEALTH TRAINING OVERSEAS

Much that has been written about the training of psychiatric personnel applies, with suitable adjustment, to other personnel in the mental health field – psychologists, sociologists, anthropologists, and so on. It is of course essential that the training needs of each of these other types of personnel receive quite specific consideration. It is harmful, as the experience of several countries shows, to regard psychiatry as the central mental health discipline and all others as auxiliary, and consequently to look upon the further training of these other disciplines as no more than a kind of diluted psychiatry.

The problem of the reabsorption of overseas trained personnel into their country of origin is more acute for the non-medical professions involved in mental health work than it is on the medical side. There are very few countries without at least some framework of organization of the medical profession, which could be adapted for reception of the returning members of the new medical speciality. But in the majority of the countries in which mental health work has only begun in recent years, there is no tradition of organization of social work or even of psychology. Thus the introduction of mental health work may entail the creation of a professional group that is entirely new to the country concerned. Formidable problems then result if, as may well be the case, no professional class exists, and if the middle classes as a whole have only a rudimentary organization or themselves are virtually non-existent. The absence of a framework to relate to causes great hardship to returning professional personnel and may hold up the expansion of training schemes for many years. With a training programme such as that described at length above, the Study Group thought that non-medical professional personnel could be more easily reintroduced to their own country if their professional role had not previously been recognized within the framework of the training institutions there. In these circumstances the new professional categories can be presented to the people of the country as an extension or elaboration of a system with which they are more or less familiar, even if it is not highly developed in their own country, and there need be no difficulties arising from infringement of vested interests or uncertainty of role.

There are many unsolved problems and much confusion concerning the roles of the non-medical professions in countries where new mental health services are developing. This point can be illustrated by the widespread adoption of the professional designation 'psychiatric social worker'. As was discussed in Chapter 9, this term originated to describe a particular style of professional orientation in the United States and a few other countries. In its now extended usage, it means many different things in terms of training, experience, and professional role. It is manifest that psychiatric social work does not present a homogeneous picture over the world, and though there may be nothing sacrosanct about a descriptive term, great variations in its usage from country to country undoubtedly lead to difficulties in cross-national communication.

When services are evolving it seems wise to adopt a flexible attitude towards professional roles, and towards the complex question of who should do what, and in what circumstances. Among the determining factors in shaping new professional roles are the educational practices in the community, the availability of personnel, the traditional social roles including sex roles, and the climate of opinion concerning public and family social responsibilities. It is often forgotten that the proper use of elaborate social services requires a relatively high degree of social integration and sophistication in the community concerned, and it is of little value to introduce a new class of highly specialized worker where the more general aspects of social work are unknown.

As a footnote to its discussion on this topic, the Study Group recorded that the personal problems of expatriate professional personnel – whether the expatriation is long term or short term, and whether it is forced by political or other circumstances or voluntarily assumed – do not receive adequate recognition, and we do not know enough about how to help expatriates with their problems.

The occasion for sending young professional people abroad for training most commonly arises when unfamiliar professional alignments or perhaps entirely new professional disciplines are being introduced into their home countries. A difficult situation may arise when, for example, a non-medical psychologist returns home to his psychiatrically underdeveloped country after a period overseas as a trainee in clinical psychology in a setting in which the respective professional roles of clinical psychologist and psychiatrist were well understood. On his return, the newly trained clinical psychologist may very probably find that his work situation is not one for which his training has prepared him. He may have to work on his own, or in collaboration with psychiatrists who know nothing about his professional skills or how to collaborate with him. Another unlooked-for outcome to overseas training is when a group of people in the home country adopt for themselves the sphere of work and the title of the returned overseas trained personnel, although they have neither the training nor the conceptual framework of the latter. A conspicuous example of this practice has already been mentioned – the adoption of the term psychiatric social worker.

Such difficulties and frustrations hinder the development of new mental health work to its optimum level. The returned trainee who cannot find an appropriate sphere of work or a professional status that satisfies him may decide that his hard work and special training are of no value to him. Not only does the work fail to grow, but no further candidates for training come forward and the whole project peters out.

If a group of untrained people take over the initiative by modelling themselves on the returned trainee and adopting his sphere of work, confusion is bound to follow. They may be excellent people, activated by the highest motives. Paradoxically, they may be capable of doing better and more appropriate work in the community than overseas trained personnel, who – as we have seen – do not invariably derive real benefit from their training. Nevertheless, their coming together as an *ad hoc* professional group offers no promise of constructive future developments. Their work is pragmatic, without unity of conceptualization, and there is wide variation in the extent of their knowledge of basic studies, which is often inadequate. A more forceful criticism is that they bring no new concepts with them; having no personal experience of alternative approaches in the field, they rely on familiar methods and traditional attitudes. They have no systematic method of evaluating past experience in terms of success or failure, and, in addition, have little to contribute to the organization of training and the building-up of services for the future.

The Study Group laid great stress on these pitfalls which tend to be associated with the organization of professional training overseas if commensurate attention is not paid to the establishment of an appropriate professional framework in the home country. Where a new professional discipline is introduced in unfavourable conditions, the development of the work to its true potential may be held up for a whole professional generation – that is, until the retirement of the pioneers, who may have been forced by the primitive conditions they encountered early on (which have long since passed and were never relevant to the work) to accept limited or inappropriate aspirations and work standards. There is also the danger that the entire concept will be ultimately rejected, because of its alien origins and the failure of cultural assimilation.

Therefore, in the planning of training schemes it is essential that the desired future professional role should be considered from the outset. Also, agreement should be sought and obtained at an early stage on standards of professional education and a code of conduct. In return for the students' acceptance of standards and codes, the community should protect a particular name or title, by restricting its usage to those who have the recognized qualifications.

Training schemes abroad are very costly, so that they should not be entered into without the fullest consideration, whatever their potential value. In most countries only a very limited number of people will be available who are suitable for foreign training, and the Study Group recommended that priority should be given to those who have already had teaching experience in their own subject, and who intend to return with the primary objective of teaching. This is the principle that has been followed in Santiago de Chile, in a training institute set up by UNESCO for the further training of people who already hold academic positions in their own country. The training institute is intended primarily for those who are already teaching sociology and social psychology in South and Central American universities. At Santiago they meet people from other countries, who, like themselves, are highly trained and, though still comparatively young, are already leaders in their professions. The Study Group would agree with the implication of this policy, that it is those who are already experienced and fairly senior who gain the most benefit from transnational training schemes.

REACCULTURATION

We have made above a passing reference to de-briefing, and to the readjustment the individual has to make upon his return to the home country after training abroad. De-briefing is a difficult undertaking and should be given serious consideration as a built-in part of any training scheme.

There are two major aspects of the realignment problem: first the returned trainee has to be freed from the 'contamination' of extraneous cultural influences to which he has been exposed during his training. That is, he has to be able to identify and distinguish the purely culturally determined aspects of his training, and make use of what he has learnt without carry-over of attitudes that belong to a quite different setting. The trainee's capacity to do this will depend to some extent upon the degree of understanding his teachers had of his cultural situation, and on their ability to help him to identify the cultural elements of the training and to make the necessary adjustments.

Second, the returning trainee has to face a change of role, from that of a privileged pupil in a foreign country to that of a pioneer working in an unprepared situation, who is required to demonstrate his usefulness to his own community before he can expect to be accepted. The trainee can be either helped or hindered in role adaptation by the attitude of his seniors and contemporaries at home towards the training that he has received, and also by evidence of knowledge and concern, or the reverse, about his country's problems on the part of the teachers in the foreign training centre.

An appreciation of these issues demonstrates the need to make stable and long-term arrangements for the training of students overseas. The day has long since passed when all that was required in order to get immediate results was the allocation of a sum of money for the awarding of fellowships. We have outlined above a model scheme for psychiatric training on the principle of bilateral cooperation. There are many precedents, relating to a wide range of subjects, of special relationships being built up successfully between training centres in one country and students in another: as, for example, between the Philippines and the United States; between many British universities and countries of the British Commonwealth; and between France and its overseas territories. Ties of language and sentiment have, on the whole, tended to preserve these special links even after independence has come. There are other examples of special arrangements growing up, largely through the initiative of a group or an individual. The University of Toronto has built up an association with Thailand, starting in the field of educational psychology and spreading to child welfare. Norway has a similar special training link with Kerala in Southern India; it started through a UN scheme to improve standards in the fishing industry in India, and has been extended to quite a wide field of social service. Where a tradition of mutual understanding and help has been established, not only do the educational needs of the expatriate trainee receive far greater understanding overseas, but also the prestige and value accorded to the overseas training in the home country greatly facilitate the readjustment of the returned trainee.

Language difficulties constitute the most serious single obstacle to schemes of foreign training; and a major disadvantage is that training opportunities in the case of newly developing countries tend to be restricted to the area of the most familiar language. Thus the old cultural ties from which the new countries have been emerging, in many cases with some difficulty, tend to be artificially continued. If they are given too much emphasis, language difficulties will inevitably reduce the training potential of smaller countries, even when they are comparatively highly developed.

Schemes for training personnel abroad sometimes encounter problems in the political sector when there is a degree of incompatibility or hostility between the respective ideologies of the two countries concerned. Where the trainee's home country is intolerant of the ideology or prevailing political attitudes of the country where the training is given, the returned trainee may find that his position has been worsened rather than strengthened by his experience. It may be that steps will be taken in the home country to neutralize the feared 'contamination' of the individual by the foreign culture.

LOSS OF TRAINEES BY JOB SEDUCTION

Training schemes of this kind are particularly vulnerable to wastage when the trainee is seduced by the manifestly greater opportunities available in the overseas country, in comparison with his own, and decides to remain there. The repercussions can be grave, especially in the case of a newly emerging country. When a government has spent money that it can ill afford in order to send promising young men and women for training to a country regarded without qualification as very wealthy and privileged, and the result is the loss of some of the home country's best brains, a negative attitude is likely to develop both towards the training country and towards the type of training it offers. If the area of training is mental health, the hostility tends to be directed to the whole notion of mental health work. On the purely practical level such incidents increase the already excessive disparity between the countries concerned, to the detriment of international relations.

Quite unconcealed attempts at this type of seduction have been reported from a number of European countries: newspaper advertisements offer training abroad in psychiatry and psychology, with student pay and the prospect of employment after training. Such harmful practices could be stopped, given goodwill, and the attention of the advertisers might be drawn to the probable ill effects of their actions on the countries of recruitment.

The trainee is subject to more powerfully seductive influences than the newspaper advertisement. The attractiveness to the foreign student of the country in which he is training is a contributory factor to the success of the training; particularly in the field of mental health, the trainee is unlikely to get full benefit from his experience unless he has a strong positive sympathy with the training country. As we have said, the student is in a privileged position, by virtue of having been selected for training abroad, and in respect of the treatment he receives as a foreign trainee. If the rosy picture of the training country that builds up in his mind is not offset by attractive career prospects in his home country, he may have little motivation to return.

Precautionary measures are sometimes taken: for example, strict conditions are laid down, stipulating that the student must guarantee a minimum period of service in his own country after completing his training. But it is difficult to enforce such conditions, which may, perversely, increase the attractiveness of the training country in the student's eyes. It would appear to be wiser to adopt a liberal attitude, giving the student freedom to work where he wishes after qualification, but before he leaves his home country and before he is subjected to the new influences, guaranteeing him a satisfying career in his home country on his return, and making quite clear to him that he is wanted and valued.

In addition to the provision of security for the trainee on his return, an appropriate selection procedure, eliminating individuals with a low level of emotional maturation, is a decisive safeguard of the interests of the home country. The student's capacity to perceive and conceptualize problems relating to the whole training situation and the extent of his insight into the needs of his own country will reveal how far he can identify with the home community and how great is the risk of his using the training for ego-centred purposes. Giving prior consideration to those students who intend to make teaching their career might be another way of arriving at the same end. One point to be watched in the selection of the more mature student for training in a foreign country is that he is not too set in his ways and culturally embedded, for this would greatly reduce the benefit to be derived from such experience. In short, the soundest way of counteracting the threat of job seduction is to make the prospect for the trainee on his return to his own country overwhelmingly attractive.

TRAINING OF RESEARCH WORKERS ABROAD

Much that has been written about professional training and the training of future teachers abroad applies equally to research workers. A distinction must be made, however, between some of the basic disciplines – such as anatomy, physiology, pharmacology, and psychology – and the applied clinical disciplines.

As far as the basic sciences are concerned, a case can be made for sending the student to the training institution with the highest intellectual and scientific standard, provided that the trainee's level of culture and command of the language are sufficient to enable him to adjust to life in that institution. In this field knowledge of the language obviously plays a decisive role. Care needs to be taken not to encourage either in the student or in those responsible for sending him the idea that pure science can be found only in a cultural setting remote from their own.

The future research worker in the clinical disciplines needs much the same conditions for successful foreign training as the future teacher and clinical worker, but in his case an added precaution is to ensure that the scientific standards of work in the training institute are adequate for the purpose.

12

Public Education for Mental Health

The success of health education in improving community standards has encouraged the hope that mental health education might be equally useful; but it is now realized that effective public education in mental health matters is a very difficult undertaking indeed. In the words of Lemkau (381):

'Public health mental hygiene is the application of the scientific knowledge about mental health and mental illness in the lives of the population served. Unfortunately, mental illnesses have been associated with mystico-religious fantasies for so long that there is a tendency, in the efforts towards the promotion of mental health, to borrow the starry-eyed enthusiasm of the fanatic reformer. In such a situation – and it is all too common – the enthusiast is likely to mount his steed of publicity and so-called public education and ride off at full speed. In doing so, he frequently wanders away from the narrow path of scientific knowledge and sets off across unmapped country, finally falling when some simple question, usually put forth by a harassed mother, looms up as insuperable because the knowledge has been left behind. Enthusiasm for a "good cause" will not take the place of scientific knowledge. To use the psychiatric jargon again, there must be "content" as well as "affect", knowledge as well as enthusiasm, if progress is to be made in mental hygiene.'

The current attitude towards mental health education, in most places where it has been attempted, is distinctly critical. It has been well stated by Ridenour (632):

'There are several lines of action to be carried out if we are to build a solid base for mental health education. We must become more self-searching, more alert to the dangers of untested assumptions, more critical of subjective value judgements. . . . To increase proficiency in judging the effectiveness of our work we must keep moving in the directions touched on in this paper:

1. Toward developing more definite criteria of validity; measures of change; controlled experiments; research.

2. Toward more careful analysis of what people want; observation of popularity, of what takes hold with the public.

3. Toward a greater degree of objectivity; learning to react as scientists, not as individuals; learning to distinguish between our own subjective and objective reactions.

4. Toward utilizing the body of knowledge derived from clinical experiences and education, systematizing it, codifying it. Examples are: knowledge about the relation of anxiety to learning; ways of interpreting unconscious motivation; the importance of emotional readiness for individuals and groups; the futility of exhortation.'

The National Assembly on Mental Health Education, held at Cornell University, USA, in 1959, agreed that the professional experts were not fully in accord about mental health education programmes in that there was a lack of clarity about goals, principles, and effectiveness of techniques. The Assembly underlined the importance of evaluation of present methods with the object of creating sounder programmes in the future.

Most recent emphasis in this field has been on community cooperation in mental health education, with the realization that this task cannot be undertaken successfully by a professional authority on its own. In the words of the WHO report on Social Psychiatry and Community Attitudes (155): 'If society is to reap the full benefit of the advance of modern psychiatry, it must learn to collaborate in the prevention of mental disorder and in the therapy of rehabilitation of the mentally ill.' In other words, further progress now largely depends on the attitude of the community towards mental patients and towards social psychiatry itself.

PRINCIPLES OF MENTAL HEALTH EDUCATION

The Conference on Mental Hygiene Practice, convened by the WHO Regional Office for Europe at Helsinki in 1959 (635), discussed the formulation of principles to be applied in educating the public in mental health matters. A key aim of educational effort was put forward – that basic mental health principles should come to be regarded by the public as common knowledge rather than as exotic dicta. Thus, mental health education programmes are likely to be most effective when they form part of general health education, which, in turn, should be part of general education, using existing educational channels. Such programmes need the backing of the appropriate authorities in the community, and should be systematically planned by experts, particularly with regard to use of the mass media; they should be aimed at prevention rather than correction, but at the same time they should be concerned with everyday problems.

At the Helsinki conference distinctions were made between: (i) programmes of mass education of the public; (ii) attempts at more individual education of those members of the community who may be in situations of stress, e.g. pregnancy or sickness; and (iii) the education of those whose mental health is particularly important to the welfare of others, e.g. mothers, teachers, nurses. Three main types of educational activity were considered: the use of small groups for clearly defined purposes; the incidental educational function of certain professional people in their daily work, e.g. in public health work; and the mass media.

According to the Helsinki conference, the aims of mental health educational programmes should include: attempts to change any attitudes and behaviour that are likely to arouse emotional problems in others; the provision of information about facilities for those in need, about the constructive handling of special problems, and about normal developmental and other phenomena; and, to some extent, the provision of information helpful to people with emotional problems.

The conference was also concerned with the special need to educate those whose occupation gave them, in practice, a public educational function. Members remarked on the general inadequacy of professional training in these regards, and on the difficulties resulting from shortage of personnel at the present time.

The WFMH International Study Group thought that its best contribution at this stage would be to discuss some of the current trends in public mental health education, without attempting to be exhaustive. A preliminary consideration is that public mental health education may be bedevilled from the start by a need to convince legislatures and authorities of the need for it. They may have to be convinced before work can begin, and it is often necessary, in order to achieve this, to try to present an image of what is intended in terms that can be understood by people who know nothing about the field.

In mental health education there are dangers in two different directions: of concentrating, on the one hand, on the mental disease aspect, with the risk of arousing the anxiety that attaches to mental illness in people's minds; and of concentrating, on the other, on modifying people's attitudes in various respects, with the risk of arousing anxiety about magical powers associated with the idea of being able to change people. The anxiety that may be built up at the prospect of a familiar person becoming different, however unrealistic or unlikely this may appear to be, can be powerful enough to close people's minds to acceptance of mental health work in any form. These two approaches are not essentially conflicting or mutually exclusive, and indeed are often combined in practice; yet most people engaged in mental health education appear to favour one approach more or less to the exclusion of the other.

Programmes of mental health education, to be effective, must be planned with regard for the individual's life circumstances and for the community atmosphere. For many years community health educators have been accustomed to seek to exert their greatest influence at times that are normally stressful for the individual; that is, at usually critical points such as leaving school and entering employment, getting married, first pregnancy, menopause, bereavement, and so on. Infant welfare workers often find that they do their best work with mothers when the mothers are encountering the normal stresses and strains associated with the bringing up of young children. It has frequently been observed that this same principle is applicable to mental health education in general, and no less to group than to individual education. When a group is faced with problems that could have been foreseen, and is finding them difficult, then, it is claimed, its members are likely to be most receptive to mental health educational work.

The Study Group was concerned with what kind of image of mental health should be put before a community in order that the work may prosper. Obviously the image would have many facets, and as many channels of communication and means of projection. We have suggested that there is no real antithesis between the approach that focuses on the elimination of mental illness, on the one hand, and the so-called positive approach, on the other. On the contrary, the two approaches are complementary, are equally necessary, and should be carefully coordinated. A rather crude illustration, however, may serve to point up the dilemma underlying such a combined approach. If a country's mental hospitals are poor and the objective is to get the legislature to spend money on their improvement, the mental health educator could reasonably be concerned to make it abundantly clear to the relevant officials just how unsatisfactory the hospitals are. A cross-section of the community, including the relatives of psychotic patients, would be likely to react to his revelations with shock and anger which could, without the most skilful handling, result in a chaotic situation that would mean the suspension, perhaps for years, of all hope of ameliorating the conditions by rational means.

There are so many sides to mental health education that the primary responsibility for its advancement will rest with different people and organizations in different countries. It is in many countries, for instance, considered to be the province of the psychiatrist; elsewhere it may be regarded as a cultural activity. In the Soviet Union mental health education is part of the function of the Central Institute of Health Education, where psychiatrists, among others, are employed as technical advisers to educators.

Some basic questions have to be answered before a programme of mental health education can be embarked upon: 'Who says what to whom? In what circumstances? To what purpose?' But the education process is more complex. Thus stated, the questions suggest that it is a matter of a simple relationship between a presenter and a recipient, a preconception that deserves examination. Not all of the many facets of the image of mental health education imply this kind of relationship, yet the questions asked leave out of account the contribution to be made by participant learning. In the mental health field this method is particularly appropriate. Examples of learning through participation include: part-time voluntary work in mental hospitals; the study of mental health problems in the community by non-professional personnel; and, as mentioned above in connexion with Taipei, the study of the epidemiology of behavioural disturbances among children, carried out by schoolteachers.

While there is a great need to expand the use made of learner participation, it is clear that for the great bulk of educational programmes more passive techniques have to be employed. Whatever the type of programme, certain points are to be noted: only those who are acceptable, culturally and professionally, to the community concerned can effectively take part in mental health education; the image of mental health that is projected has to be acceptable too, and not regarded as foreign; a clear distinction has to be made between the presentation of what is generally accepted fact and the reporting of what is no more than minority opinion. In order that such educational work may continue and develop in the community it is prudent for promoters not to overlook the education of legislators. Programme planners should also be alive to the favourable effect of counselling and clinical services on the receptiveness of the community to mental health education. Thus to ensure that the personnel of the clinical services are aware of their potential contribution is itself an important part of the education programme.

TECHNIQUES OF PUBLIC MENTAL HEALTH EDUCATION

Are there useful roles to be undertaken in the mental health education of the public by specific bodies, such as WFMH in the international sphere and national mental health societies more locally? The Study Group was inclined to agree with those who feel that the usefulness of many of the usual educational activities – e.g. the provision of literature on mental health practices, group discussions, lecture courses, and so on – is limited because of the vague generalities that are necessarily involved. It might be more valuable for educational programme builders to devote attention to the organization of series of seminars, in which experts in various disciplines and cultures could discuss the principles of mental health education in the presence of representatives of those who were to carry out the educational campaigns.

Schoolteachers have a leading role in mental health education. They are commonly among the first people in the community to be singled out for such work, but the therapeutic aims implicit in mental health education may not prove entirely helpful to teachers. The teacher who is laudably engaged in attempting to deal with mental hygiene problems in his class may be less useful as a teacher to those who do not require his therapeutic aid. It is probably more valuable to help teachers to recognize the commoner forms of emotional disturbance in children and to ensure that they know to whom to refer the individuals concerned than to complicate the teachers' role and place a burden of therapeutic responsibility on their shoulders.

In the more highly developed countries the multiplicity of agencies in the health education field is an advantage to mental health, on the whole, though there are dangers of overlap and unprofitable competition. It is widely held that it is better that health education generally should be sophisticated in regard to mental health than that mental health education should be easily identifiable as a separate process – however sophisticated. This view is becoming more generally accepted. For example, in Taiwan today, no mass media or other specific means are employed in mental health education; instead, teachers, general practitioners and the public health service carry out such programmes in the course of their ordinary duties.

The presentation of material in mental health education is a complex undertaking. In our view, the first essential is to communicate the material to the public in a well-organized form, which will facilitate recognition of its relevance and significance. Usually, at the outset of a programme, the ignorance of the public is profound, and unconscious resistance to knowledge is so easily roused that indirect or subliminal methods are generally ineffectual. Thus new ideas have to be presented to the people in terms that are already familiar to them, which may involve breaking up material that appears to the expert to be indivisible. How to present mental health material through the mass media while avoiding sensationalism has yet to be discovered. This is one of the reasons why emphasis is placed on the so-called positive approach, with the objective of strengthening the tendencies towards health rather than of stressing the angle of mental ill health.

We have referred above to the difficulty of bringing about a reform of mental hospital conditions without publicizing their shortcomings, and thus, in turn, discouraging people who have personal or family problems from seeking help. In addition, publicity about poor conditions in mental hospitals can be quite inimical to attempts to secure a more favourable attitude, on the part of the public and of the potential employer, towards mentally ill people living in the community and, particularly, towards patients discharged from such hospitals. The educators are faced with a dilemma: if they claim that the discharged patients are as sound and well as anyone else, then the community cannot logically be asked to give them special consideration; and if they underline the fact that the patients have been ill and are in need of help, then the acceptability of the latter to the community or to employers is bound to be reduced.

If mental health education is putting it across to the public that mental hospitals are bad and in need of reform at the same time as it is seeking to change public attitudes towards mental hospital patients, it can hardly occasion surprise that in fact public attitudes towards mental hospitals harden and ordinary people feel increasingly sceptical about individuals who have been unfortunate enough to be treated in such places. Yet most programmes appear to focus on the shortcomings of present treatment methods and only a minority attempt to rely extensively on a more positive kind of approach. The growth of positive methods is much hampered by lack of more precise knowledge.

Whatever type of approach is employed, it is generally agreed that mental health education cannot be effectively carried out merely by telling other people what to do, a procedure that is of very little use in any counselling activity in this field. The task of the mental health educator can be epitomized as that of presenting the facts in a form that the recipient can appreciate, and then helping him where necessary to draw his own conclusions.

Further study should be given to the technique of communicating research findings and recent advances in knowledge to the wider public, and to the separate but equally necessary matter of how to mobilize informed opinion in relation to current problems. Both types of activity are more effectively carried out where there is a recognized channel of communication between the communicators and the public, such as might be provided by a mental health society. Indeed, experience has shown that the mobilization of informed opinion can be accomplished successfully only within the recognized channels of influence within the community. The engagement of public opinion is a polymorphic matter, because it may reasonably be held that there is a potential mental health angle to all activities involving people. We feel that it is not too far-fetched to remark as an illustration that even the activities of morticians might constitute a mental health problem if, for example, they encouraged for commercial reasons certain activities in relation to the dead – embalming rituals, displays of mourning, and the like. At least it may be readily agreed that morticians can both contribute to and reduce the wellbeing of their living clients. Such issues are all within the range of mental health interest.

The second objective, the communication of more scientific findings to the general public, can, in comparison with the mobilization of public opinion, be achieved successfully by more remote means, since the intention is to give information to a recipient body rather than to secure its assent or its active cooperation. An example of successful communication on this basis is the Report of the WHO Regional Conference on Mental Hygiene Practice in Helsinki (102), to which we have made extensive reference. The material of this report was prepared by an interdisciplinary international group; it was found to be widely applicable, and has been appreciated and drawn on in many parts of the world. The WFMH study of *People in Hospital* (259) is another report, prepared by an international interdisciplinary group, which has aroused widespread interest, at least in those countries where the provision of hospital services is more than a series of emergency arrangements.

An unsolved technical problem concerns the definition of the appropriate level for the communication of scientific knowledge – not too popular to risk distortion, and not too highbrow to limit circulation. It is essential to note that any form of educational material that is not presented to the recipient in his native tongue may suffer a critical loss of effectiveness. In the case of small countries whose language is understood, spoken, and read by relatively few people, there may be a serious poverty or restriction of educational resources. These difficulties call for an international organization to be responsible for the translation of works from their original English, French, Spanish, Russian, or German into less widely used languages and, conversely, for the translation of material from the lesser known languages into the more commonly used languages to promote its more general distribution; and to subsidize publications in language areas where sales are small. An international organization with adequate financial support and resources could make a really significant contribution to mental health education in these ways.

COMMUNITY LEADERS

We have referred frequently in this volume to the special needs of people holding responsible positions in a community, such as teachers and other community leaders. We have advocated a separation of the therapeutic role from that of the mental health educator, at least in schools, but it is nonetheless important that teachers and other community leaders should be fully aware of the mental health work that is being undertaken in their community, and particularly of the mental health significance of their own activities. In order to bring this about, the conceptual structure by which people understand the nature of their contribution to mental health in the community needs to be improved. This, it is felt, will be more successfully achieved by participation methods than by didactic information-giving.

It is not necessarily true that the community leaders and teachers provide the most useful starting-point for an attempt to make an impact in mental health work in a community; each community should be considered individually. Whoever is involved in the education process, however, should strive to awaken to the full the interest and capacities of the learners themselves, and to remember that the classical method of clinical teaching by pathological example may generate considerable anxiety among the taught. Anxiety so aroused can be used constructively to improve the quality of the learning, but if it is not skilfully handled it can seriously distort the total picture gained by the student and reduce his capacity for understanding.

THE MENTAL HEALTH SOCIETY

The most widely distributed instrument of mental health education is the mental health society, at the time of writing found in forty-six countries. The roles and functions of mental health societies are discussed more extensively in Volume III of the current series, *Mental Health in the Service of the Community*, and here we shall make only a passing reference to their part in mental health education. This is clearly a key function of mental health societies; indeed, Krapf (378) states that their main function is an educational one, and in his view the only propaganda that convinces is 'the adequate presentation of facts'.

When a mental health society operates at a national level, its most obvious means of communicating to the public is through the national press and other mass media; it also communicates directly to members of the government. A regional society will have a similar role in a more restricted area. Local mental health societies, however, are different, in that their members are actually living in the community and are under observation. Their most useful role is to concern themselves with the practical problems of the local community and with personal issues, and it may be that the degree of success that attends their educational efforts will be highly related to the effectiveness of their contribution to the solution of the problems they encounter.

TECHNIQUES OF LOCAL MENTAL HEALTH EDUCATION

It may be suggested as a basic principle that those who undertake mental health education in a society should work in close co-operation with those who understand the methods of education that are effective in that society. However, it would not be sensible to ignore accumulating knowledge of how other people learn in many different kinds of society. Hence an open mind should be kept as to the suitability or unsuitability for mental health purposes of other people's educational practices, wherever they may be found.

Another basic principle is that the teaching method and the material that is being transmitted should be linked together so intimately that they constitute a unity. It is axiomatic in teaching theory in this field that a distinction cannot be made between the subject-matter, on the one hand, and the technique for putting it across, on the other.

A third principle is the need, in every educational programme, to observe precisely what is actually being learnt. It is well recognized that there is not necessarily a simple correlation between what the teaching agency is putting out and what the recipients are in fact learning. In illustration of this point an educationist in the Study Group cited an example sometimes used in teacher training in order to provoke discussion: during a classroom lesson in mathematics perhaps 15 per cent of the children are in fact learning some mathematics in a creative way, in other words, getting to know how to apply mathematical principles, and about 15 per cent are learning simply to do the sums; perhaps 30 per cent are learning to dislike mathematics, and another 20 per cent are learning to dislike the teacher; 10 per cent are learning to dislike the whole set-up of school; and 10 per cent are learning nothing at all. A similar situation would be found in the context of mental health education.

It may be inferred from the foregoing discussion that the Study Group considered that mental health education programmes should always be worked out in close cooperation with the educators in the society in which they are undertaken, but should also take account of relevant educational principles, wherever they occur. A wider question arises in that active educational methods imply relationships between teacher and taught, and it is relevant to inquire whether certain relationships in the learning situation might themselves be inimical to mental health. Some educational systems or situations give rise to, or even foster, the development between teacher and learner of relationships that inhibit learning and increase the learner's anxiety. Only the most general comment can be made on this point, since there is no opportunity to make a detailed study of relationships in a given society.

It may be useful briefly to discuss some aspects of the question of authority in education in general terms. First, a clear distinction needs to be made between 'authority' and an 'authoritarian attitude' in education. The giving of certain information with authority relates to the need of the individual to whom it is given to trust the source of the information, whereas an authoritarian attitude adopted by a teacher derives from his personal need.

This point is particularly relevant to the case of people who are emerging from life in the kind of traditional society in which authority has counted for a great deal. There are many things in traditional societies that are done in a particular way for no reason within the experience of the members currently living in the society. Although questions of the law and its interpretation may be decided upon by lengthy discussion in the councils of the society, matters of habit or custom are more usually passed on without examination.

For example, in the upbringing of a child in a traditional society, many things are done in a particular way and in no other way, and the correctness of the traditional practices remains unquestioned. When families move from this kind of society to a city, the women who are mothers of young children experience certain new anxieties because they encounter a variety of attitudes and practices with regard to child-rearing – artificial feeding, for instance, and manufactured baby foods which circumstances may compel them to use. The attitude of these mothers towards feeding and handling their children, which was previously one of unquestioning conformity, becomes one of potential anxiety and worry. The effect of their changed situation is pervasive. A newly migrated town family may have come from a farm where the mother was accustomed to tell her child to go and play outside; in the new dwelling on a busy street the same instruction, given unthinkingly, would expose the child to mortal danger. Again, the migrant families may have belonged to a society in which the mothers were, by tradition, obsessional about their children's bowel movements. As a result of changes in living practices and diet in the new surroundings, the regular bowel habits of some children may break down; cases have been described of mothers applying quite traumatic devices in an attempt to restore the accustomed routine. In such circumstances it is hardly useful to argue with the mother the pros and cons of different procedures, because she has not been accustomed to exercise choice in matters of custom and habit. The only basis on which the mother might be expected to cooperate effectively is to be told what she should do – as she would have been had she visited the tribal medicine man, however irrelevant or impossible to follow his prescription might be in the altered living circumstances. Therefore the reasonable recourse for the adviser is to assume whatever authority he can and affirm that it is harmful to the child to treat him in this way. Then the mother should be given a set of simple instructions, obviously appropriate to the current living conditions and easy to follow and put into practice. Only as the level of education of the mothers rises, and particularly as they gain confidence in their ability to manage things in the new environment, are they usually able to get insight into the whys and wherefores.

In other words, the nature, quality, and values of the culture are the first considerations in planning new forms of mental health education. Where the culture has been authoritative and traditional, a suitably tempered approach should be adopted, even in stages of transition, in preference to a non-directive counselling type of approach that may be appropriate to more sophisticated cultures.

The above example oversimplifies the problems involved in moving directly from a traditional rural to a new city culture, because it does not allow for the probable fact that that city culture is itself in a process of rapid change. Indeed, it is very common in the world today for whole subcultures to be subjected collectively to rapid and radical change, so that mental health educators must be concerned with what kinds of educational approach are appropriate to a generally changing situation, as well as with what are fitting for a specific culture. There are many different ways in which education can be presented: in terms of reward and punishment; in automatically self-rewarding situations; through the use of authority and authority figures in the culture; or in terms of prestige in relation to other cultures. It is often possible for children to serve as an incentive to their parents' learning, as in the case of rapidly changing societies when adults may be able to accept a change for their children that they would not accept for themselves. The degree of usefulness of these various ways will vary according to the culture, but they all need to be related to the common factor of change if they are to be successful.

A further factor to be taken into account is that in all but the simplest societies some kind of hierarchical organization develops in the education system. There are likely to be two opposing influences in operation: on the one hand, the style of teaching used by the people at the top of the hierarchy will tend eventually to reach the latest comers at the other end of the educational chain; but, on the other hand, if the village schoolteacher or the public health nurse or other fieldworker adopts a certain fixed method of working, this rigidity may work up the hierarchical scale in due course, along with the promotion and increasing seniority of the worker. In a rapidly developing social organization, the first fieldworkers are almost certain to receive the fastest promotion to high positions. Thus, in a traditional society, if the pioneers are allowed to employ, unchecked, the uncritically accepted methods of instruction that were mandatory in the society's past history, the organizational foundations may be laid for a type of authoritarian educational method which is incompatible with change, and which may endure throughout the professional lifetime of the pioneer generation.

It may be conceded that comparatively little is known about the whole question of education for change, but certain things are becoming clear. For example, attempting to instruct people on how to adapt to unfamiliar situations by formulating items of new behaviour in rigid terms is a poor preparation for change, perhaps even worse than permitting them comfortably to pursue their old traditional behaviour. An anthropologist remarked that a study in the USA had shown that behaviour newly learnt from external sources may be maintained even more rigidly in a state of continuing change than traditional customary behaviour, unless the learner is enabled to recognize that the new behaviour may be impermanent. This may be achieved by some formulation in the individual's mind as, for example: this is what we do now; but tomorrow, or next week, or in another city or country, or when the children are older, or when we have a hospital, things may be different.

There have been innumerable instances, in many countries,

where the result of accepting new social practices from outside sources has been rigidity, and this is particularly true of such matters as infant-feeding practices, health measures, and educational techniques. Where precisely defined practices that resemble a cult rather than a scientific operation have been successfully introduced, they tend to be rigidly adhered to and quarrelled over indefinitely. It is a universal experience that it can be immensely difficult to get people to see how much of human behaviour is governed by temporary fashion rather than by unquestioned and unquestionable law.

An apt illustration at this point is provided by the attitude of a young Polynesian: he had set up a school in an island village, on his own initiative and according to what he thought a real school should look like, although he had had only two years of schooling himself. When congratulated on his very real achievement, he said: 'Don't call this school. If you call *this* a school the government won't send me a real school. I am only keeping the children's minds clear until the school comes.' It must have been a common experience in countries where mental health work has been started that progress has been blocked in certain directions for a professional generation because of the early enthusiastic and rigid adoption of half of an ill-understood idea that has had to die with the generation that introduced it before more genuine development has been possible.

CONSONANCE WITH CULTURE

The complex question of the cultural relevance of mental health education cannot be disregarded. A few comments will illustrate some of the complexities. For example, it has been reported that in some English-speaking countries a greater response can be obtained by using the term 'emotional' health in preference to 'mental' health. Apparently the notion of emotional disturbance evokes less anxiety than that of intellectual disorder. Moreover, it is common experience that better results are obtainable if the field of activity is narrowed down to certain selected sectors of the public, and, in particular, to professional and semi-professional people. It seems likely that in most places the selection of specific fields of activity and of media of communication will be largely determined by cultural factors.

A difficulty that has been reported in English-speaking countries, and may also be met in others, is that the mental health programmes that secure the most financial and influential support are not always those that, professionally speaking, would be given a high priority. In the present state of public education the conditions that have the greatest financial appeal appear to be those involving a visible physical handicap, whatever the mental or emotional difficulty. In some countries it may be the case that those who control public finance have a disproportionate if indirect influence on the programmes of mental health organizations, because the promoters of mental health activity naturally tend to apply for funds for programmes in which they know that the financial administrators are interested. This situation amounts to a key problem of mental health education, because wherever financial administrators have the power to discriminate between alternative proposals and to decide which to support, it follows that the future direction of mental health work may be indirectly determined by people who have no special knowledge or experience in the field, and it is therefore a primary task to attend to their mental health education.

Difficulties may also arise in those countries in which it is common practice for wealthy individuals, personally or through foundations that they have endowed, to support programmes of research or new work. In some cases it has become customary for the government or public agencies to leave this type of activity more or less entirely to private organizations. Thus the situation can, and does, arise in which an executive of an influential foundation – who may have no training or experience in any of the sciences of human behaviour, or no advanced scientific education – is in a position to prevent, without realizing what he is doing, the development of the most promising of new ideas; or to insist on the continuation of work methods that have outlived or never proved their usefulness. In these countries, among the key people and community leaders towards whom mental health education needs to be directed at the outset, are those officers of governmental and voluntary agencies who, through the financial power that they wield, can promote or destroy initiatives in mental health work in the community.

We would re-emphasize the need to tie in mental health education programmes with significant factors in the cultural situation over a wide field. For example, in some societies it may be found that no progress can be made in mental health education until certain acute social problems, such as housing or unemployment, have been dealt with. Not only programmes but techniques need to be related to local values; for instance, the quality of the reputation and the use made of the mass media in a certain community might make them quite unsuitable for mental health education purposes; or, again, the attitude towards authoritative and didactic teaching methods could make such methods either ideal or useless for mental health education, according to the given culture.

In short, mental health education programmes must be designed to grow in with the general cultural situation, so that any changes that are hoped for as a result of the programmes will be grafted into the particular society as a living part of it. What have come to be widely regarded as the standard means of mental health education – lecture, public meeting, film show – can no doubt be effective in any society with a good level of literacy and general education; but their value is immeasurably reduced if, as too often happens, there is inadequate or haphazard preparation. In some areas these methods could be worse than useless, and we suggest the WFMH might consider the question of what general educational principles and specific techniques could be applied with validity to various types of cultural situation. To give an example, it has been suggested that in the United Kingdom television is the most effective single medium of health instruction, and the printed word and poster advertising are more or less unavailing. It would be valuable to know to what extent, if at all, this is true, both there and in other countries.

In the present state of knowledge, precise statements cannot be made about the value of different techniques in relation to cultural influences. We have only vague generalizations, such as that: in the United States the group discussion method is in favour; in India, the words of the religious teacher tend to be more noticed; in tribal organizations, the opinions of the chiefs are given more weight; and so on.

Finally, we would draw attention to another unsolved problem, that of assisting the public in the difficult task of reconciling its sometimes conflicting obligations: to have a scrupulous regard for the civil rights and liberty of the individual; to ensure the proper discharge of the community's responsibility to protect mentally ill patients from the effects of their own actions and vulnerability; and to safeguard the interests of third parties.

13
Public Education and Mental Health Problems

INDIVIDUAL ANXIETY AND MENTAL HEALTH EDUCATION
The Study Group agreed that while it would certainly be a major aim of mental health education to alleviate inappropriate or excessive anxiety among the public it is well to recognize that there is such an entity as reasonable or healthy anxiety, which must be distinguished from what is unreasonable and unhealthy. As has already been noted, it is healthy and indeed a condition of survival that human beings should be concerned to ensure that they have an adequate food supply. It would certainly not be a task of mental health educators to help people to become less anxious about possible starvation in a country where there was in fact a shortage of food. On the other hand, for a citizen of the United States to be seriously worried about his own possible starvation would be an irrational anxiety and a fit subject of concern to the mental health educator.

There was considerable discussion in the Study Group as to whether it was legitimate – or even possible – to attempt to alleviate anxiety by authoritative pronouncements. The Group did not come to any agreement that this could be a satisfactory educational technique in this field. Members thought that mental health issues are so complex that they can only very rarely be resolved into simple authoritative statements; and that any attempt at definitive pronouncements that were other than clear and authoritative would tend to increase rather than decrease the amount of irrational anxiety borne by the less-well-educated part of the population. It is extremely difficult to decide precisely, on the one hand, what are indisputable facts that can legitimately be put forward in authoritative form; and, on the other hand, what are areas of discussion that must be given a non-authoritarian type of presentation because they are not incontestable. It was remarked that it is not uncommon for a statement to be made with an assumption of great authority that serves only to make it clear to the hearers that the speaker is not at all sure of the truth of what he is saying!

Where accidents, cancer, and addiction to alcohol, drugs, and tobacco are concerned, health educators customarily attempt to stimulate a response by playing upon fear and pity. It appears to us that such motivation can rarely enter into mental health propaganda in a crude or unsophisticated way, because of the destructiveness of the anxiety that is thus aroused; nevertheless, we might profitably consider whether it could be useful in our field to seek to rouse anxiety deliberately for educational purposes, by more refined techniques.

We have already referred to the dilemma that faces the promoters of mental health programmes of how to get the public to realize that the mental hospitals are bad so that more money may be forthcoming to improve them, without destroying their confidence in the efficacy of the psychiatric treatment that is available and thus discouraging members of the public from seeking specialist help at an early stage of difficulty. This kind of dilemma is not confined to mental health work, but is common to many educational activities, even at a scientific level. Much discussion of learning theory has centred on the role of anxiety and stress in learning.

In some ways, would-be mental health educators have contributed to this dilemma, in that, like the drug firms – the manufacturers of medicines for the relief of headaches, lassitude, insomnia, and so on – they have at one and the same time attempted to draw the attention of the public to the severity of various disorders and to the availability of various anodynes and remedies. Indeed, the comparison might be taken a step further, for it might be argued that the old-fashioned custodial type of mental hospital is no more than an anodyne for the social disturbance sometimes caused by the psychotic in the community; and that its function may be justly compared with that of an alkaline powder in the treatment of dyspepsia – the removal of disagreeable sensations from consciousness.

Just as the drug manufacturers may have a great deal to answer for by the creation, through their advertising, of neurotic attitudes and psychosomatic symptomatology, so some mental health educators may unwittingly have stirred up anxiety by directing the public's attention to the search for an immediate cure, instead of to the more time-consuming objectives of identifying root causes and achieving genuine prevention. A public brought up to look for gimmicks and remedies may well become too anxious to have patience for a search for origins.

Even in the case of learning by children in school, the role of anxiety is ill understood by a high proportion of educationists, particularly those who fly to immediate punishment for learning failure and who give an unthinking allegiance to that strange pseudo-principle of 'spare the rod and spoil the child'. It is but a commonplace observation nowadays that it takes a relatively small exposure to anxiety to reduce a child's capacity for rational control and action, and therefore his learning capacity, and that, though children vary widely in these respects, the general threshold of anxiety tolerance is very low indeed during childhood.

We are convinced that there is a great need for a more objective study of the use of anxiety in educational measures in the mental health field. In much of the world among ordinary people there is a raised level of anxiety due to changing ways of life. As more and more people become separated from the support of traditional circumstances and values, and are subjected to experiences of change that are beyond their control, the factor of anxiety in adaptation to change becomes increasingly important. We believe that a balanced and reasonable perspective in these matters includes the realization that, under conditions of general and radical change, complete freedom from anxiety is no less morbid than excessive anxiety. Charcot once remarked that it is not normal to be normal in abnormal conditions.

In a world in which there is much to be anxious about, it is clear that it is easy to overestimate the possible dangers of mental health programmes, and it is prudent to retain a realistic view and especially not to be too sensitive to the anxiety-raising qualities of films and similar activities. It is quite certain that if mental health workers do not undertake these educational measures for themselves others will, perhaps for reasons of seeking commercial advantage. That there is a great market for advice in personal problems is revealed by the amount of space devoted to this type of activity in the daily press and journals. The field is wide open for exploiters as well as educators, and we feel that mental health interests have a responsibility in this field that it is dangerous to underestimate.

The Study Group thought that some of the anxiety that appears to be aroused by mental health educational programmes may in fact be displaced from more deep-seated anxieties concerning changes in family relationships and population movements that are part of a wider spectrum of change, but in this instance are projected upon the mental health educator as a result of his having brought these matters more sharply into the public consciousness. However, this possibility increases rather than decreases the responsibility of the educator to ensure that the educational material does not create more anxiety among the recipients than they can tolerate without losing some of their capacity to learn effectively. It is the sum of anxiety, including that which has been displaced from the personal problems of the individual, that has to be recognized and taken into account, together with the likelihood that people of different cultures, or of different social groups in the same culture, differ in the level of anxiety that they can tolerate while still being able to learn.

We would emphasize that the fact that learning may be inhibited by anxiety must be appreciated by those initiating programmes of education in mental health. Many devices and techniques have been advocated for turning aroused anxiety to positive account in the learning process. For example, it is sometimes advocated that lectures and films, and even radio and television programmes, should never be arranged unless the recipients are given the opportunity for group discussion of the contents of the programme immediately afterwards; it is difficult to see how radio and television features could be included in such a ruling. The idea behind this argument is that group discussion will enable the abreaction of anxieties and tensions raised by the programme, so that the recipients' emotional involvement can be put to constructive use. We believe that a skilfully handled discussion may well serve this purpose; on the other hand, where group discussion is undertaken more or less fortuitously, the sudden awareness of their common bond may actually heighten the anxiety of the group members, without their realizing that such anxiety is widely dispersed throughout the population, or virtually universal. The Study Group was of the opinion that where literate populations are concerned greater use could effectively be made of the more personal and less collective effect of the written word read in private.

Many empirical methods have been proposed for dealing with anxiety in the interests of mental health. There is widespread realization of the need to understand the potential effects of anxiety, as was illustrated during the Study Group's sessions on this topic from the experience of a psychiatrist who had served in a military medical capacity in World Wars I and II. He reported how, during the First World War, the phenomenon of shell shock became widely recognized in the Western European theatre of war, and its origin came to be understood through the psychological treatment of casualties. Shell shock was shown to be, broadly speaking, a severe state of conversion hysteria due to attempts to repress fear rigidly – greatly reinforced by old and universal military traditions. A considerable change of attitude was brought about in military circles in a number of countries subsequent to the war. For example, a Commission in the United Kingdom recommended that all members of the armed forces should be taught to regard fear and anxiety as normal phenomena in situations of danger; to recognize that there was something wrong with the man who did not experience them, and that what really mattered was how the man did his job in spite of his fears. In World War II it could be claimed that, where soldiers had been trained in this way not to be afraid of their own anxiety, the incidence of conversion hysteria was dramatically reduced. In contrast, where the old attitudes still prevailed, in general, conversion hysteria was not less prevalent than previously. This is an example of how mental health education, properly applied, can have quite remarkable effects.

THE ORDINARY PERSON AND MENTAL HEALTH PROBLEMS

A large part of the complexity of mental health education can be attributed, as our discussion in the earlier sections of this volume has shown, to the fact that the concepts of mental health and mental illness vary so enormously and in very subtle ways between individuals. There is a remarkable poem by Louis MacNeice[1] which, though not written with this aim, could be said to express some of the speculative attitudes that the ordinary person might feel when approached by a mental health educator:

> *Goodbye, Winter,*
> *The days are getting longer,*
> *The tea-leaf in the teacup*
> *Is herald of a stranger.*
>
> *Will he bring me business*
> *Or will he bring me gladness*
> *Or will he come for cure*
> *Of his own sickness?*
>
> *With a pedlar's burden*
> *Walking up the garden*
> *Will he come to beg*
> *Or will he come to bargain?*
>
> *Will he come to pester,*
> *To cringe or to bluster,*
> *A promise in his palm*
> *Or a gun in his holster?*

[1] *Collected Poems, 1925–1948* (London: Faber & Faber; New York: Oxford University Press).

Will his name be John
Or will his name be Jonah
Crying to repent
On the Island of Iona?

Will his name be Jason
Looking for a seaman
Or a mad crusader
Without rhyme or reason?

What will be his message –
War or work or marriage?
News as new as dawn
Or an old adage?

Will he give a champion
Answer to my question
Or will his words be dark
And his ways evasion?

Will his name be Love
And all his talk be crazy?
Or will his name be Death
And his message easy?

A central task of mental health education is to help people to recognize when behaviour is indicative of mental ill health. How can the ordinary person, without special experience or education in this field, learn to discriminate between behaviour that suggests the presence of some disturbance that requires treatment and behaviour that could be reasonably anticipated, given the cultural circumstances? What is at stake here is the bringing of cases that need attention to the notice of the therapeutic agencies at an early enough stage to give them a good chance of a successful outcome.

Two broad fields of work are involved: first, a programme for the education of ordinary people, and especially of young parents, to help them to distinguish between what they need to seek advice about and what they can deal with themselves. Naturally, specific cultural phenomena will have to be taken into account, and programming will be a more complex undertaking in the case of cultures in the process of change. In a society in which the traditional customs are unbroken, an individual child's deviation from the expected patterns of behaviour, when not responsive to the normal corrective pressures, may have greater pathological significance than a similar amount of deviation in a child in a society where there is normally a range of permitted or expected behaviour for both parents and children.

The second educational field is that of helping clinical workers – public health doctors, nurses, and social workers – to recognize from mothers' statements about their children, and from their own observations of mother-child interaction, the earliest indications of disturbance. Sometimes such indications may be concealed beneath what passes for normal or desirable in that society. For example, in the United Kingdom it is a commonplace to hear a mother remark with satisfaction: 'My child never cries'; or, less commonly but not infrequently: 'My child is so good that sometimes, when I have left him by himself in a room, I peep in after a bit to make sure he is all right, because I never hear a sound.' This mother may feel thankful that her child is not a perpetual troublemaker and attention-getter like her neighbour's child, whose behaviour she may regard as being indicative of a bad upbringing or a difficult or spoilt child. Yet clinical experience of child psychiatry suggests that a noisy attention-getting child may have a better outlook in the future, in terms of personality development, than a very quiet, over-good toddler.

Similar illustrations may be found at other phases of child development. A psychologist remarked that in some countries teachers are becoming more discriminating in their attitudes to the range of children's behaviour they encounter and, for example, no longer set such a high value on good, conforming behaviour. It is by no means universally held nowadays that sustained un aggressive conformity is to be preferred to more socially troublesome conduct, in respect of the future mental health of the child;

although very many schools are still conducted on the old assumption.

Comparatively little is known about this area, and not only is far more research needed but also a greater dispersal of knowledge among professional people and others who handle children. It is particularly desirable that the diagnostic skills of people with professional training in mental health work should be more readily available in schools and in other spheres of public work with children.

There are numerous difficulties in the way of securing early and reliable recognition of mental trouble and of the significance of disturbed behaviour, by responsible people and by the public generally. We shall discuss in Volume III of this series the danger that an individual may become quite wrongly labelled as suffering from a disease – a misfortune for the individual no less severe than that his difficulties should go unrecognized because of a lack of agreed simple criteria of health and disorder which can be taught to non-professional people. Again, the transference of criteria of health and sickness from one culture to another without due modification can have equally unfortunate results. Clinicians are familiar with the way in which mistaken conclusions can be drawn when psychological tests are used in cultures other than those in which they have been standardized. Another common error is to arrive at a diagnosis of mental deficiency from the results of intelligence tests administered to children who are living in poor material conditions, without adequate nourishment, and, an even greater handicap, in cultural and educational poverty.

A psychiatrist reported to the Study Group the findings of an investigation in the United States concerning the attitudes of people, including some who might be regarded as potential patients, to psychological difficulties. In a study of a national cross-sectional sample by social science techniques, one subject in four said that he had had worries or problems sufficient to make him think he might be having a nervous breakdown, and that professional help would have been of some use. Only one in seven had sought such help, and the distribution of this seventh was influenced by age and by level of education. The commonest source of help sought was the clergyman, with the family physician second, and the mental health (or psychiatric) agency third. It was also found that people who lived in communities where there were active mental health agencies and educational efforts sought help much more readily and to a greater degree (from all sources) than people who lived in areas where there were no such provisions. This finding appeared to be independent of whether or not the individual actually knew of the existence of clinical facilities in his community. It seems to have been a general and indirect result of mental health educational work.

INDICES OF DIFFICULTY OR DISORDER

The early recognition of cases needing help depends on the ready interpretation of indices of difficulty by professional people, parents, and relatives, and it is an urgent prophylactic measure to increase knowledge of what indicates failing mental health at all ages. The Study Group stressed the need for widely ranging studies in this area, to include, for example, processes of following back from a case which has broken down in order to discover the aetiological factors, and those of following forward from a situation conceived as potentially harmful in order to find out what happens. There is a distinction between these two procedures, which can be illustrated by reference to United States studies in the field of delinquency. Repeated studies of juvenile delinquents more or less confirmed in delinquent behaviour have testified to an abnormally high incidence of broken homes among this group. On the other hand, follow-up studies of children from broken homes have consistently failed to reveal a higher proportion of delinquent children than control studies of children from unbroken homes. This latter finding has sometimes been interpreted as indicating that a broken home is not significantly associated with delinquency; but the studies do not throw light on the total measure of social difficulty in the two groups. It is legitimate to suggest that the explanation of these apparently antithetical findings could be that the broken home indicates a situation in which individuals are liable to become vulnerable to the influences that result in delinquent behaviour.

Clinical evidence suggests that the concept of the broken home may need to be interpreted more broadly: not simply as the absence of a parent, but to include disturbance or disruption of the network of human relationships that is normal for the culture in respect of both the family and the neighbourhood group. This wider frame of reference might facilitate a breakthrough of knowledge in this field. (In this connexion it is suggestive that a recent study of post-partum psychosis in the United States showed that its incidence was systematically related to whether the mother's mother or a sister or close female friend lived within a radius of one hundred miles. It was also associated to some degree with the type of housing area in which the young family were living, and especially with whether the young mother had any friends of her own generation in the area.)

Studies of this kind indicate ways in which it might be possible to develop indices of incipient mental health difficulties, for instance, by directing attention first to the types of community where trouble might be expected to arise on theoretical grounds – for example, new towns; new suburbs; areas where there are migrants who do not speak the language of their new country, and young couples who have moved out of range of parental support or away from relationship networks. Thus the prophylactic focus would initially be the location of those communities and social situations that appeared likely to give rise to difficulties, and less attention would be given at first to the identification of the individual at risk. An advantage of this approach is that it avoids attaching a stigma to an individual who is conceived of as being especially at risk, by the very attention that is meted out to him.

In recent prophylactic work a similar principle has been applied to the case of the individual child in the home: attention has been focused not so much on the visible aetiological factors that have led to the child's difficulties as on the specific qualities of the home situation that may have rendered the child vulnerable, in terms of inadequate parent-child relationships, temporary or part-time separation, the presence of handicap, and the rest. Thus a mother's inability to give herself wholeheartedly to the nursing of her baby, although the home may be very adequate as regards other expressions of affection and care, could be a more serious indicator of potential difficulty than the fact of a broken home or evidence that the parents are on bad terms. In the last case it often happens that one parent is able to give the child what he needs for healthy relationship formation.

An anthropologist pointed out that this situation-oriented approach to the prevention of the formation of difficulties has been anticipated, in a sense, by the *rites de passage* found among primitive societies in respect of conditions in which people are especially vulnerable: e.g. the menarche, marriage, bereavement, the puerperium, or when a man has killed another man, etc. In such *rites*, the whole community is mobilized for the protection of the individual. Learning from this example, it might be a valuable objective to create such *rites de passage*, in a more scientific sense with the use of modern sociological techniques, for vulnerable individuals.

As a postscript to our discussion on indices, we would emphasize that our concept of an index is not that of a phenomenon that exists in its own right; rather, we use the term in the sense of an indicator of the existence of a certain state of affairs, whatever interpretation the observer may put on it. In other words, the object of identifying indices is that they may draw the attention of observers to a state of vulnerability in the individual that may develop into a more serious condition unless protective mechanisms are mobilized.

READINESS TO CONSULT THE SPECIALIST

The question of indices is intimately bound up with public recognition of the proper role of the mental health specialist in these matters and public readiness to consult the specialist. Public attitudes towards the mental health specialist are revealed to some extent in the use of euphemisms – 'nerve specialist', 'neurologist' – and also in some commonly held stereotypes: that he is a superhuman know-all with powers of divination; or a 'head-shrinker' or 'trick cyclist'; or a foreign-looking and foreign-sounding individual, with neither sense of humour nor common sense; and so on. A social psychologist remarked that there is some evidence in the United States that there are wide class and ethnic differences in attitudes to psychotherapy and in readiness to go to a psychiatrist. These are related to other stereotypes, such as the expectation of receiving drugs from the doctor and the dissatisfaction when they are not forthcoming.

On the other hand, the work of Shirley Star (666) and others in the United States has indicated that negative attitudes to psychiatry and psychiatrists are by no means universal, and may not even be widespread. The psychiatrist is in a fairly high position in the prestige hierarchy of the general American population and, to a greater or lesser degree, in other countries too. But wherever he stands it can hardly be doubted that stereotypes of the mental health specialist and attitudes towards him are highly pertinent to the progress of prophylaxis as well as treatment.

CONTINUING NEED FOR
POSITIVE MENTAL HEALTH EDUCATION

It is a truism, frequently repeated, that whenever ordinary people set out to think or talk about mental health they succeed only in considering mental disorder; and, in general, it is found that the public is seriously misinformed about these subjects. We have considered modern concepts of mental health at length in Chapters 7 and 8. Here we shall return briefly to review popular concepts of mental health in connexion with public education.

In a recent work based on techniques of opinion polling, Nunnally (644) claims that the American public that he sampled is not misinformed, and that it holds very few misconceptions. He finds that there are some areas in which people are relatively uninformed, but in general they turn readily to experts for guidance and accept the latter's authority. However, this author seems to have no doubt that mental disorder is stigmatized in the public mind with a general 'negative halo' that includes the patient, the treatment methods, and to some extent the experts themselves. A further point made by Nunnally is that experts have extremely conflicting views about the materials suitable for public education in mental health. The Study Group considered that, owing to the specific nature of the techniques employed in his study, Nunnally's findings should be accepted only with reservations; they would not be generally applicable even in the United States to those sections of the population less well educated than the sample studied, and especially not in other countries, where attitudes might not be at all comparable.

There can be little doubt that mental health lacks a positive image in all parts of the world. It is reasonable to infer that the increasing numbers of people who are coming for earlier treatment in many countries may indicate a lessening of fear about the major mental illnesses; but the slow growth of public insight concerning the significance of lesser conditions and the psychosomatic field generally shows that the position is far from satisfactory everywhere. In fact, acute embarrassment is being caused to mental health work in many countries by the consistently hostile attitude of the press and other organs of opinion to any measure involving a more liberal attitude to mental disorder, and by the strong tendency in the public mind to link mental disorder and other abnormalities with crime and antisocial behaviour.

In a working paper, MacKeith pointed to the strong unconscious factors that determine popular attitudes to sick people and to their treatment. Sigerist, in *Civilization and Disease* (669) and other writings, has attempted to distinguish between attitudes to physical and mental illness respectively, and to acute and chronic illness, and has also suggested that the different attitudes depend on unconscious as well as conscious emotional forces. Main (668) has drawn attention to the unconscious ambivalence of public attitudes to mental hospitals and to the people working in them, and in his work on epilepsy as a social problem Cohen makes the same point (330).

Similar unconscious factors, MacKeith noted, may be involved in the stigma that attaches in varying degree, not only to mental illness and epilepsy, but also to leprosy, tuberculosis, venereal disease, and skin diseases generally. The influence of these unconscious factors has been discernible also in some places where the introduction of greatly improved mental health services has in some ways tended to reduce as well as boost public confidence. Where comparatively minor psychological disturbances are treated by dramatic, even traumatic, methods, and where a rapid turnover of hospital cases involves members of the community more in the acute phases of illness, public anxiety may increase and reinforce unconscious resistances already there. The practical implications of the role of unconscious factors for the design of programmes of mental health education are self-evident.

After reviewing the literature in this field, Ahrenfeldt came to the general conclusion that public attitudes to mental illness are much influenced by cultural differences, which largely determine the question of acceptance or rejection of the sick individual and the concept of what constitutes a mentally disordered or deviant individual. Public attitudes are also influenced by educational factors, and by official policies in regard to mental health services, availability of psychiatrists, and so on.

One of the less widely recognized effects of the stigma of mental disorder is that closely related and cognate fields tend to be neglected by research workers because there is a resistance in the public mind to any hint of a connexion with mental disorder. Thus, hitherto, problems of alcoholism, sexual promiscuity, crime, and delinquency have rarely been studied adequately from the point of view of mental disorder. The reason may be a taboo due to fear of the inference that a psychopathological approach implies an attempt to remove asocial, antisocial, and delinquent behaviour from the field of personal responsibility. The Study Group took the view that social pathology may be as significant to mental health studies as public health morbidity is to medical studies in general, quite apart from the converse usefulness of knowledge of psychopathological processes in the understanding of behaviour.

There is not uncommonly a strong undercurrent of resistance to objective investigations into mental pathology in connexion with social studies, and it is interesting to note in this regard that an interdisciplinary Institute of Criminology, the first of its kind in the United Kingdom, was recently established in a university (Cambridge) that had no clinical medical school and no chair of psychiatry, and had shown relatively little activity in the field of the social sciences. The greatest strength of the new Institute appears to be on the legal side.

No less resistance is found to the carrying-out of studies of retardation in development using a sample representative of the whole population, possibly in part because families fear that by being included in the investigation they may attract something of the stigma that attaches to mental deficiency. Scientists are unanimous in their view that a great deal can be learnt from reliable longitudinal studies of children and their families, but their objectivity is liable to be impaired by the resistances that we have referred to and by the activities of pressure groups of parents of handicapped children. These resistances and, indeed, the activities of the pressure groups have to be skilfully handled in the furtherance of mental health educational programmes.

14
Other Mental Health Educational Methods

Studies have been made of many areas when clinical facilities were being introduced there for the first time. It has been the usual progression of events that a clinic is established before public demand for its services has arisen. The impetus for the new venture usually comes from a group of professional or other sophisticated people who learn of the success of clinics in other areas. Once its work has begun, an efficiently conducted clinic almost invariably creates an increasing demand for its services.

Many attempts to establish clinical services have been hindered in the early stages by a vicious circle – as long as no services exist the need for them is likely to pass largely unrecognized in the community; while the need remains unrecognized there is little likelihood that the community will support an attempt to provide the services. Another pitfall to be avoided by promoters is that a vigorous programme of education may make a section of the community aware of the need for clinical services before it is possible to make adequate provision, with the result that such services as may be improvised are grossly overburdened and thus appear to be ineffective. The community is then left with the dual impression: first, that the whole situation was largely artificial – that is, that the attempt to provide services itself stimulated a demand for them which would not otherwise have arisen; second, that the services are ineffective and do no good, anyway. Reactions of this kind have set back for years in many countries efforts to introduce special services for maladjusted and delinquent children and for various clinical and educational problems.

The public educational work of clinics has sometimes been deliberately promoted: for example, local welfare groups have been encouraged to take some initiative in early case recognition. It is a controversial issue that is likely to have varying success in different countries. In Victoria, Australia, a widespread attempt has been made to utilize the services of voluntary groups interested in the care of the mentally ill. Out of a population of three million people, about half a million voluntary workers are involved. Their activities are many and various, and some of their best work has been in the aftercare of patients discharged from mental hospitals.

It was reported to the Study Group that there is a considerable body of informed opinion that is not in favour of clinics' undertaking health education work as a separate activity; rather, it advocates the fostering of a health educational element in every contact between the physician and his patient, from the earliest instance. This view appears particularly applicable to the mental health field.

We need to consider more carefully the possible influence that the patient under treatment, and after treatment, can have on the reputation of a mental health service and on the attitudes of local people. The effect can be negative, as is illustrated by the harm that was done to the reputation of psycho-analysis during the 1920s and 1930s by the behaviour of some analysands, and by the unbalanced enthusiasm of some patients who attempted to carry psycho-analytical ways of thinking into their social life. On the positive side, the moral effect of a cure on the community is undoubted; and even if a cure is not fully complete many ex-patients have had enough insight to set up a chain reaction leading in the direction of greater tolerance and understanding of ill people among their acquaintances.

In addition, there are many indirect effects to be considered. For example, if a young woman consults a doctor about her senile parents, then the way in which the doctor handles the situation, and his behaviour towards the parents and towards the young woman herself may influence her behaviour in later different situations, possibly with her own children. The doctor may also help to create an image of senility in the young woman's mind, which may affect her own behaviour when she becomes old. The

Study Group made the general point that the stereotypes that a community holds about what is meant by mental health are largely derived from the experience of patients and relatives as they attend clinics, and that both clinical and lay staff are often too immersed in their immediate task to spare a thought for the image that they are themselves creating. We all know of instances when harm has been done to public attitudes towards mental health by clinic procedures that have been adopted without thought for their more public effect. Thus the old-fashioned neurological clinic, in which a patient with a hysterical conversion symptom was first demonstrated to students as presenting a functional malady and then cured by suggestive magic, was the worst form of mental health propaganda. It seems likely that the more modern sessions of electroconvulsive therapy in hospital outpatients' departments, conducted with similar lack of thought for the patient's personality and his relatives' reactions, are no better as propaganda.

The Study Group was fully convinced of the positive support that could be won for new mental health services if they were effectively demonstrated at the outset to people who had previously been without such facilities. The first impression that a new clinical service makes is quite a decisive factor in the degree to which it will succeed in a community.

The WHO Expert Committee on Mental Health (155) observed in 1959:

'As increasing numbers of the community come into contact with patients who have been successfully treated, attitudes based on fear and hopelessness are likely to be superseded. It therefore follows that a basic necessity for improving community attitudes towards mental illness is an extension of active treatment facilities closely linked with the community. The two processes are thus seen to be interdependent: better treatment leads to improved acceptance of the mental patient, and increased public tolerance is needed for further advances in social psychiatry. An important principle to be kept in mind is that specialized activities in the field of mental health should be integrated, or at least closely coordinated, with other general health services. Thus, treatment for the mentally sick should be made available in the same way as specialized treatment for the physically sick. This should help to convince the public that mental illness is just as susceptible to treatment and cure as is physical illness.'

From a review of the literature in this field, Ahrenfeldt concluded that there is reason to believe that popular attitudes and prejudices about mental health matters are modifying appreciably, if slowly, in many countries. In the United Kingdom in 1957 the Royal Commission (404) noted:

'There is clearly a strong feeling among the general public . . . that many patients who are now certified could be given the treatment and care they need without certification . . . While there has been a general increase in public sympathy towards mentally ill patients and a wider understanding of the fact that mental illnesses are . . . usually susceptible to treatment . . . certification seems to have attracted to itself the prejudice and misunderstanding which at one time surrounded the whole idea of mental disorder. It is often thought to imply life-long mental instability, or to carry a social stigma both for the patient and for his family which may persist even after the patient leaves hospital, and to cast doubts on his mental or even on his moral reliability throughout his life, and perhaps on the mental stability of his children and other near relatives.'

On the other hand, in the United States, the Joint Commission on Mental Illness and Health, in its Final Report in 1961 (389), stated:

'Repeated exposure of the shameful, dehumanized condition of the mentally sick people who populate the back wards of State hospitals does not arouse the public to seek sweeping humanitarian reforms. . . . It has been the special view of the mental health professions that people should understand and accept the mentally ill and do something about their plight. The public has not been generally moved by this protest. People do feel sorry for the mentally ill, but in the balance, they do not feel as sorry as they do relieved to have out of the way persons whose behaviour disturbs and offends them. . . . The fact that society tends to reject the mentally ill is, of course, well known; little significance seems to have been attached to it, however.'

It is not intended to evaluate these two statements; they are merely reproduced here by way of illustration. To take another example, it is interesting to note that in Peru, where there is a remarkably high prevalence of convulsive disorders, the general population show 'frank cultural rejection of epileptics' (63). But in England (where the prevalence of epilepsy is appreciably lower), it has been similarly recorded that:

'The public have long cherished the belief that epilepsy is synonymous with mental deficiency and uncontrollable criminal impulses . . ., and the epileptic is thus too often treated as a pariah. . . . Another unhappy outcome of the general ignorance and misrepresentation of epilepsy is the sense of guilt which it kindles in the parents, and which unless they are reassured may lead through mutual reproach to domestic strife, which reacts adversely on the child' (330).

The WHO European Conference on Mental Hygiene Practice in Helsinki 1959 (635) stressed that public health nurses, properly trained, are in a favourable position to help in many of the psychological aspects of the problems they encounter. For such help to be effective, however, it is essential that mental health principles are more closely integrated into public health practice, and that concern with the emotional problems surrounding illness is regarded as within the scope of a public health nurse who, on her part, must be able to recognize and deal with these problems incidentally, in such contexts as they arise. Examples are mothers' anxieties about their sick children; husbands' anxieties about their pregnant wives; and patients' anxieties about their own illnesses.

This conference noted that, to enable the patient to understand the public health nurse, some simple explanation and discussion may be necessary, in the course of which, if she is to play her part effectively, the public health worker needs to be aware of the existence of emotional defences, and how to deal with them. It was felt that the public health nurse should limit herself to the more practical matters and act strictly in the context of the patient's physical illness; that information should not be forced upon people who do not ask for it but, when it is asked for, the information given must be reliable and reassuring. The conference was clear that the giving of gratuitous advice on domestic and family matters should be avoided, but nurses should be in a position to tell the patient or relatives how they can get expert advice, particularly on those matters about which the nurse herself is unable to be reassuring.

MENTAL HEALTH EDUCATION IN SMALL GROUPS

Many mental health educators regard group discussion as their most valuable educational method, whether the groups consist of patients themselves or of the parents of children at guidance clinics; and whether they are conducted by public health workers, teachers, the police, the clergy, and so on, in their respective spheres of action. The Helsinki conference (635), in emphasizing the value of these techniques, insisted that mental health educators today must be competent and experienced in managing small discussion groups. In principle, the conference recommended that all group discussion topics should be geared to the needs of the group, which entails some care in group selection to ensure that a range of values and attitudes, representative of the community, is provided for. Awareness of the existence and nature of different social attitudes is particularly required in cases where the management of children is being discussed. Whether the method is accepted by the group will depend to a large extent on the behaviour and language of the educator. Other points made by the conference were: information given to groups must always be reliable and certainly never misleading; even correct information may sometimes need to be withheld from groups because of the emotional misunderstandings it may arouse; all information dealt with in groups must be understood by the members, hence the importance of discussion; educators who take part in discussion group activities must be competent in the field of group dynamics.

THE RELEVANCE OF
MENTAL HEALTH EDUCATION TO SCHOOLS

Hardly anyone would contest today the usefulness of some more or less formal or systematic mental health education to all whose professional vocation brings them closely into contact with people. There is less agreement about when such education should commence, and it is a noteworthy fact that mental health and human relations subjects are, with very few exceptions, not taught in the schools of the countries about which we have had information.

It is not uncommon where pre-school children's groups exist – nursery schools, play groups, or more casual social groups – for children to be directly taught some kind of human relationships technique. Such teaching efforts are rarely systematic: they often depend on what adults feel about how children ought to behave; but their common objective is to enhance the understanding of one child for another, so that children may show consideration for each other. Thus the basic lessons of social conduct – not trampling on the rights of a weaker child, sharing adults' attention and material goods, taking turns, encouraging generosity and discouraging greediness, and so on – may be taught by direct means.

In countries with compulsory primary school education this kind of teaching is not usually given in the schools proper; or perhaps it would be more accurate to say in this connexion that modes of conduct and social codes are presented to the children as rules to follow, and not as pieces of dynamic behaviour to understand. Thus, questions of human rights and personal relationships and so on may become obscured by social practice and caught up in the taboo systems.

One of the great difficulties in effecting changes of attitude in this area is that it is not until children have matured, and not until they have passed through the conventional control of behaviour usually taught by schools to a stage at which they can consider human relationships in a more sophisticated way, that they are able to learn about and understand human dynamics. It it probably not unrealistic to remark that, even in sophisticated societies, perhaps the majority of adults never get appreciably beyond the conventional control of human behaviour into its understanding; and that those who do develop further usually do so on a basis of developing their own theories of psychology if they have not been trained in any of the schools of psychological thought. Usually they have no basis other than their individual capacity for empiricism on which to formulate their principles.

The teaching profession up to now has not started out with any particular advantages over other educated members of the community in respect of knowledge of the psychological determinants of behaviour. It follows that a major reason why so little has been done about mental health and human relations in schools is that so few teachers themselves possess any organized or systematic knowledge of this field. They, like other people, proceed on a rigid basis of convention, modified in some cases by empirical experience. There is perhaps a circular mechanism in operation here, in that the teachers' own systems were probably developed and became rigid while they themselves were still at school, and, apart from very minor modifications by later experience, particularly during their comparatively brief period of training, their early-formed conventions have tended to be reinforced by their immediate return to the school atmosphere. In other words, it is only too easy for conventions governing behaviour and human relations to be perpetuated automatically in the school from generation to generation.

The Study Group concluded that the primary mental health education objective in this connexion should be to introduce into schools a greater degree of conscious consideration of the principles underlying items of behaviour. But in order to do this it is clearly necessary to secure among the teachers more awareness and more objective examination of these matters, which, in turn, calls for a comprehensive programme of mental health and human relations education of teachers, both in teachers' training colleges and in the early days of their professional career.

In the case of the younger children in junior schools, our view is that the subject of human relations is best introduced somewhat indirectly by bringing to the forefront of the children's intellectual notice some of the basic points about communication. To illustrate the sort of thing that would be suitable for this age of child, we might cite the imparting of simple facts, e.g. that what one understands by another person's behaviour is not necessarily what that behaviour means, nor even what that person is trying to convey. This kind of lesson could be presented by means of simple dramatic techniques of role-playing and charade. As for where it would fit into the school's time-table, it is obvious that there would be difficulties in any educational system that adhered strictly to a tight curriculum rigidly divided among scholastic subjects.

At secondary or high-school level the objectives would be very different, and the methods might range from adaptations of the usual techniques for teaching science to a sophisticated use of the humanities to further human understanding. Thus, general science programmes could include simple laboratory experiments on learning, for example, using some of the standard techniques of psychology courses through which the more neurological aspects of psychology are introduced to the student. By such means, also, an elementary knowledge of reflexology could be acquired. Again, in the study of chemistry and physics, students are well used to discussing the properties and reactions, including the dynamic qualities, of matter. Why should they not also consider the dynamic properties of human beings? In biology, which has become increasingly popular as a school subject in recent decades, there is still a strong tendency in many countries to restrict interest to the morphological aspects, but there seems no reason why morphology should not be taught in terms of animal behaviour, so that from a critical study of animal behaviour the student may be better placed to evaluate human behaviour.

Other school studies can be involved – we have referred elsewhere to the way in which classical literature can be used to introduce students to the principles of human interaction. A great deal is done at present in many schools to make character studies along these lines, but they are not always effectively related to the day-to-day experience of the children. The teaching of history lends itself to interpretation with psychological insight, but is also prone to distortion or, at least, unreliable interpretation because of political or nationalistic bias. The subject of geography, whose boundaries are extending in schools, seems to be an ideal vehicle for introducing the child to the elementary principles of ecology, sociology, and human group relations. An appreciation of other subjects, such as logic and statistics, could be gained from school courses more frequently than it is at present – to great advantage, since two of the major obstacles to the mental health education of the public are a general poor capacity for logical thinking and the almost total inability of the ordinary person to handle numerical data critically. Greater competence in these areas could make inhabitants of the modern world much less vulnerable to 'admass' pressures.

Thus a great deal of psychology and human relations could be introduced into school courses in indirect ways that might be expected to have an optimum effect. In addition to such indirect approaches there are certain aspects of mental health education that are suitable for direct presentation to children. It might be difficult to find an appropriate label to add to the curriculum to describe these areas of study: 'psychology' is obviously inappropriate, and the term 'humanity' would be liable to be confused with 'the humanities'; 'behaviour study' is another suggestion. In essence, the aim would be to increase understanding of ourselves. The courses could incorporate something of what is now taught in schools under the heading of civics or citizenship, though as commonly presented these subjects are mainly concerned with structure and form. The real focus of study would be the more intangible aspects of human relations. There seems no reason why, as a result of a year's course, high-school children should not get a grasp in principle of such matters as unconscious motivation, and begin to understand the nature of tradition, prejudice, discrimination, and so on. Some aspects of group behaviour could be examined, and individual and group defensive reactions to anxiety and guilt. In the complex field of psychodynamics the learning process would have to be kept at a simple level, with the main objectives of stimulating in children a healthy curiosity about the whys and wherefores of human behaviour, of implanting in them the desire to know something about why they feel as they do, and of engendering the realization that they need not accept behavioural phenomena uncritically at their most obvious and manifest level.

A considerable amount of attention has been given, without entirely satisfactory results, to the more explicit teaching of psychology and the social sciences at a level immediately below that of college. In the United States efforts to develop this aspect of teaching have led to the introduction of human relations as a set subject in high school. The view was expressed in the Study Group discussion that to a non-American observer it might appear that the impetus to such teaching in American high schools arose from the national need to inculcate a sense of nationhood in a comparatively large immigrant population; this would also explain why any specific proposals in favour of similar teaching have made little impression in Europe. Such a view would suggest that what is aimed at in these teaching programmes is the encouragement in the children of a certain pattern of behaviour; whereas the Study Group was thinking rather in terms of the kind of educational reform for which progressive educationists all over the world have been working for many years, namely, that of bringing into the classroom increased understanding and insight with regard to human relationships. It might fairly be said that traditional teaching of the humanities has been explicitly concerned with this kind of objective, though perhaps not at the level of conscious awareness that is now being sought.

The success of such innovations is dependent on a supply of schoolteachers who have the necessary degree of sophistication. As remarked above, most people have no more than an empirical psychology of their own to work on, so that without much more formal training, little headway can be expected in the introduction of human relations angles in schools, under whatever name. In the first place, therefore, efforts need to be directed at teachers' training colleges in order to create an interest in this dimension of education and a demand for its inclusion in school curricula.

In the course of discussing the training of teachers in mental health principles we remarked on the fact that increasing proportions of children are coming into organized education all over the world, intensifying the need for teachers' training in the field of human relations. Another point to be considered is the future effect on society of an increased understanding of human relationships deriving from new developments in education. We need to know more about the contribution of education to social change, especially when society is in a state of rapid development. It can hardly be doubted that there are tremendous social implications whenever the educational system of a society is expanded with great rapidity and on a big scale.

The Study Group was impressed both by the potential contribution and by the complexity of this area. With a view to stimulating a more scientific spirit of inquiry into these issues, it was recommended to WFMH that an investigation be started of how children at different ages and in different cultures develop their notions about other human beings, about human nature, and about psychology. At the same time, it would be valuable to make a critical survey of past attempts to introduce psychological material into schools, with the objective of improving techniques and discovering how it may best be done.

One factor that complicates the teaching of mental health and human relations in schools is that the processes of maturation among schoolchildren are far from homogeneous. Precise data are not available, but it may be generally true that those students who are going on to higher education tend to develop relatively slowly on the emotional side in comparison with the rapid rate of their intellectual maturation. Conversely, young people who leave school early in order to go to work may achieve a relatively greater degree of emotional and social maturity while remaining more limited intellectually. Since the teaching of human relations, whether by direct or indirect methods, perhaps depends for its success more on emotional than on intellectual maturity, the attempt to deal with these matters in schools may lose effectiveness because of the variety of levels of maturity among the scholars. We need to know far more than we do at present about optimal ages for different types of learning experience among children of different levels of ability and maturation. For example, we do not know whether the optimal age for the understanding of human relations varies according to degree of intellectual ability.

On one aspect of mental health in schools, opinion appears to be deeply divided, namely, the role of teachers in the therapy of disturbed children. This matter has been carefully studied in some countries, particularly in the United States, and in many places versatile services have been built up to help disturbed children, variously called school counselling, school psychological service, and so on. Most people would agree that in principle teachers ought to be able to recognize disturbance in children, and therefore need to know what to do about the problems they discern, and to have precise knowledge of channels of reference. But there is little support for any suggestion that teachers should themselves assume a directly psychotherapeutic role with children under their care. Again, it is generally agreed that teachers should be capable of handling a certain amount of emotional disturbance in the classroom, as a function of normal interpersonal relations between teacher and pupils. Ability to get the best out of disturbed children and to prevent and forestall incipient disturbance is extremely valuable in a teacher, but many teachers who are very able in most other respects may have little skill in this area because of personality reasons.

PARENT EDUCATION

In recent years parent education and parent-teacher cooperation have been widely advocated, but the movement has developed only patchily and only in a few countries. In the United States educational system it is now standard practice to have a parent-teacher group, responsible for its own programme, attached to the school. Many schools have specially appointed counsellors on their staff to look after the psychological and social welfare of the children. In Sweden, too, parent-teacher cooperation has grown into a nationwide organization, *Malsmännens Riksförbund*, which publishes an excellent monthly journal for parents, called *Barn* (*Children*). In France, *L'École des Parents et des Éducateurs* in Paris has shown similar initiative and has been instrumental in stimulating comparable groups in a number of European countries. In the United Kingdom there are associations both of parents and of parent-teacher groups in many parts of the country, but beyond a general encouragement at Ministry of Education level, there has been little attempt to create a national movement.

A recent international survey by Stern (640; see also 636, 637, 639) notes some of the high hopes that have been pinned on parent education: that it will add to the most productive years of adult life; that it will help in the solution of certain social problems, e.g. hostility, prejudice, criminality, mental disorders; and that it will make a constructive contribution to public health, child welfare, and education. Stern observes that although the impression created by parent education is favourable, no objective studies have been made of its value, and to remedy this deficiency, the Paris conference on research in parent education has planned a number of detailed investigations. Stern also remarks:

'Experience has shown that *laissez-faire* methods, a hit-or-miss approach, an occasional burst of activity and other unplanned efforts are not effective enough. The educational help is not available when and where needed. If parent education is to advance beyond the enthusiastic local effort and individual initiative, some stable organization is needed. .... At the present time, the danger of casual indoctrination through media of mass communication – in the absence of any recognized service – is greater than the risk of indoctrination by a service which has to answer for the information and advice it gives. As long as no organization can claim a monopoly and the usual democratic safeguards are included, the danger of indoctrination is reduced.'

COMMUNITY DEVELOPMENT

A good opportunity for the advancement of mental health education, and one largely neglected, is presented by the planned community developments that are being carried out in many countries. They are undertaken for various reasons. In the older industrialized countries with dense populations, the problem commonly presents as one of population overspill or movement of industry. In the less developed countries the aim may be to accommodate expanding populations in areas that have been thrown open as a result of increasing technical resources. It is a commonplace experience today for whole new cities to be created in a space of ten years; in the planning of these cities great care may be taken over siting, layout, communications, supply of public utilities, design of buildings, public health measures, etc., but only rarely is the life that the community will lead there made the subject of serious reflection. Many of the older industrialized countries have had unfavourable and unfortunate experiences through creating new single-class communities dependent on one specific industry. Another common form of social development that has had and is having harmful effects is that of the transient working community, which no one regards as home and everyone wishes to leave as soon as economically possible.

The Study Group was convinced that a great deal can be contributed to human happiness by applying modern sociatric skills to the planning of new communities; and by using modern technology to fit new industries to existing communities rather than attempting to create new communities *ad hoc*. One can hardly overstress the educational gain that a community derives from experiencing a successful evolution into a new style of life, as compared with the disruption of human relations that occurs when a community is destroyed and aggregated elsewhere amorphously.

MENTAL HEALTH EDUCATION IN DEVELOPING COUNTRIES

The Study Group briefly considered the question of mental health education in countries where there is no developed concept of public welfare responsibility or action, and where there are specifically local and traditional ways of handling conflict situations and social problems. It is not always recognized that the sociological and biological factors operating in societies that are underdeveloped in this sense may be no less complex than those in the more developed communities.

In the training of people for mental health work in rapidly developing areas, it is a common practice to employ basic principles which are known to be valid for countries that are more developed in these respects, in the hope that students who are well versed in their own cultures will be able to select for themselves the useful parts of the teaching they receive. However, it may properly be argued that it would be better to find out how cultures differ before attempting to transfer educational methods. From a knowledge of the culture of a country as a whole, those aspects more favourable for mental health education could be identified and employed in promoting changes, and, as the society moves to new ways of living, it would be possible to ensure that the changes advocated were appropriate to the particular culture at the particular time.

It is usual for a culture to feel the first impingement from outside as much in the educational sphere as in any other, and although the foreign influence may tend to be destructive of local custom, its impact in the educational area may be conducive in the long run to mental health in the community since it may help children at least to change with the times.

In general, the changing patterns of family life now in process in much of the world have tended to reduce the prominence of the tradition-directed personality (512, 570, 667), and have increased the variation in pattern between one society and another. If a society is changing in ways that make it more like a so-called Western society, then the techniques pertaining to the latter become more useful to mental health education than the traditional teaching practices in that society; but techniques have to be adjusted to the state of development in the region as a whole as well as to the stage reached by particular communities.

It is impossible to discuss such a wide and varied subject in a narrow compass, and we shall add here only a comment in principle. The Study Group referred to the confusion of thought that has gathered around the nexus of ideas concerned with the tradition-directed personality and its implications for education. Much of the confusion lies in the commonly held concept of the traditional teaching pattern in many cultures, by which the pupil receives straight information without discussion, and raises questions only for elucidation. Perhaps too much attention has been concentrated on so-called authoritarian methods of teaching and not enough on the real point, which is not the method of the teacher but the quality of the participation of the learner. Currently, the term 'authoritarian' is frequently used in a pejorative sense in order to devalue the type of relationship that is based on the authority of one party and the recognition of that authority by the other. In fact, this situation has been and still is characteristic of teacher-pupil relationships in very many types of learning situation all over the world, but it is not justified to assume that the giving of information by one party precludes participant learning.

Whether or not participant learning takes place may be determined largely by the conditions in which the teacher and learner operate together, and among the decisive factors is the state of the learner's mind, his readiness and preparation. There are some common situations in which the pupil can learn most effectively by taking certain pieces of information on trust. This is true in the main of the process of induction of principles, because no pupil approaching a new subject is in a position to establish the veracity or otherwise of each item of information that is presented to him as a fact. Circumstances compel him to take a certain amount on trust, at least for the time being, until he has achieved a sufficient degree of organization of the subject-matter to be in a position to examine the principles critically for himself. However, even when the pupil has learnt effectively by accepting, in the initial stages, the validity of the material, there should come a stage in the learning process – in that same subject – when he is no longer able to react in this way. When that point is reached, either the pupil will tend to reject information he has not checked for himself or it will make no impact on him and will not result in action.

Thus the question of whether information is given straight or whether other methods are used, involving a more practical approach and a greater degree of participant learning, is best decided after a more complete analysis of the educational process. An analysis of objectives is especially desirable when it is proposed to apply a technique evolved in one country for a similar purpose in another. As an educational psychologist remarked, it is more pertinent to discover how the process of education is carried on in the society it is intended to help than to attempt to import into that society ideas based on educational processes in one's own society. For example, it would be generally acknowledged that the misuse of authority has inhibited a great deal of learning in what is known as Western society; this does not justify the assumption, however, that, because traditional learning methods in India have been based even more firmly on the authority of the teacher than Western methods have been, authority in education is likely to inhibit learning in India also. Nor would the mental health educator be justified in assuming that, because the learning process in India depends to a large extent on the spiritual authority of the teacher, therefore mental health education should be presented exclusively in a similar fashion. There are, of course, other learning traditions in India in addition to that of the Guru and his disciple, of which the village tradition of the elders in council is but one. The issue is complex and calls for attention.

The Study Group came to the conclusion that the essential prerequisite to the application of mental health education methods in a culture where mental health studies have not been previously explicit is a complete analysis of cultural attitudes to the existing learning and teaching situation and practices. Only with this kind of preparation can educators be flexible in their approach and avoid the formation of misleading stereotypes about teaching and learning, especially in relation to the largely false antithesis between so-called authoritarianism and learner participation.

15
Use of the Mass Media
in Mental Health Education

The use of the mass media – by which we mean the national and local press, journals and magazines, pamphlets, radio and television, posters, advertisement hoardings and illuminated signs – is a highly controversial issue in the field of mental health. In 1956 the findings of an investigation into some problems in this field were published by the American Psychiatric Association (648). Among the sample population studied, it was found that in the area of opinions and common knowledge there was a clear relationship between 'correctness' or factual basis of opinion and educational level. This suggested that it is reasonable to convey simple factual information by relatively direct methods of communication at a level appropriate to the education of the recipients. On the other hand, the investigators found no indication that simple educational methods are effective in respect of public attitudes towards mental illness. They concluded that we do not know what sorts of new experiences, methods of education, or media of communication would be effective in order to change public attitudes in this area.

Among the dangers to be faced is the widespread dissemination of a seemingly ineradicable misunderstanding of key principles, a classic example being the public attitude to the findings and teaching of schools of psycho-analysis on the sex instinct. It might almost be said that psycho-analysis has been misunderstood by the general public in as many ways as there are reactions to human anxiety, and at every level and type of education, including psychiatric education. A recent, pointed example of misunderstanding has been in the reception of Bowlby's work on the separation of babies from their mothers (407). What these studies have, in fact, contributed to knowledge might be summarized briefly in the following way: they have established the objective fact that when babies are separated from their mothers for significant periods within a certain age range, some of them show lasting evidence of having suffered trauma. Later work still in progress is beginning to indicate more precisely which babies are vulnerable and some of the ways in which the harmful effects of separation can be prevented, or mitigated when they have occurred. This work has aroused a great deal of anxiety among people in many parts of the world, more or less irrespective of the kind of organization and functioning of the families involved. On the one hand, it has been reported that some parents now feel overwhelming guilt if they are separated, however briefly, from their children. On the other hand – and perhaps as a reaction against the manifest irrationality of the conclusion that the attitude of these parents implies, namely that all babies suffer lasting harm if separated from their mothers – other people have rejected the whole notion that babies *may* suffer when separated. Where either or both of these misunderstandings are prevalent in a locality, the anxiety aroused may effectively neutralize the value of Bowlby's findings, which are among the most valuable of recent scientific discoveries for purposes of public education.

The Study Group felt that whenever controversial topics – such as child-rearing – are the subject of public education work a clear distinction must be maintained, in the presentation of material that is found to arouse emotional reactions, between what is given to the general public and what is used for discussion in a narrower context among the professional workers concerned.

RELATIONSHIP BETWEEN PRODUCER AND CONSUMER

There is a growing body of professional opinion that the mass media are most valuable for public education purposes in the mental health field when they can create and form part of an ongoing relationship between the producer and the consumer. Examples are the regular advice columns that appear in many newspapers and magazines; the Study Group agreed that there is good reason to believe that much of the work in this field is undertaken by journalists with a sense of serious responsibility. There is plenty of evidence that the columnist becomes a familiar and trusted figure to his regular readers, and it is also claimed on his behalf that any anxiety that is aroused can be controlled to some extent by private correspondence between the columnist and the reader, in which the columnist attempts to provide a personal service. We have strong reservations about the wisdom of attempting to discuss in the advice columns of newspapers and magazines a selection of clinical or real-life problems sent in by readers. This was an earlier feature of the activities of these columnists, which is now not so common. The inherent difficulties are considerable: for example the columnist cannot know for certain whether he is dealing with the personal problem of the inquirer, and it is extremely probable that the situation is presented from the highly subjective viewpoint of the inquirer and oversimplified. In attempting his answer in public, the columnist cannot even guess at the complex motivations of the people concerned who are unknown to him, and the effect of his blind reply on parties to the dispute or problem who may recognize the situation – or erroneously think that they do – could be disastrous. There is no reason to suppose that he will do good rather than harm. It seemed to the Study Group that this whole area has not been sufficiently explored: its dangers are not perceived, and its potential for good not fully realized.

A good example of the establishment of a relationship through the regular issue of bulletins on mental health topics is provided by the *Pierre the Pelican* series (641), prepared by the Louisiana Association for Mental Health, for parents of new babies. The public health authority sends letters to parents at stated intervals, starting as soon as the pregnancy is notified and continuing for about two years. The letters are distributed approximately monthly, and each deals with the kind of situation that the parents may be expected to be facing at the time. The report of the Cornell meeting (633) stated that this series 'appears to meet most of the accepted canons of communication theory'. The main danger that might be foreseen from such activities is the setting up of rigid and not necessarily appropriate standards of expectation of babies' development in the parents' minds; this could result in an increase in anxiety among those parents whose babies are not conforming to the common pattern.

Organizations that have established an ongoing educational relationship with the community are in a position to make effective use of single issues. For example, two special issues of the WHO periodical *World Health* (May/June 1959 and July/August 1961) which were devoted to mental health, did, we understand, effectively present to an interested, if limited, section of the educated public in many countries a great deal of basic information about mental illness. Another excellent example of a different type was the production by Guy's Hospital, London, of a 'comic' designed to give information to children going into hospital and to their parents (293) – again, a highly selected and personally involved 'public'.

Radio and television differ in several respects from the printed word as channels of mental health education. They are mass media, but they operate in the home in a far more intimate way than does the printed word. There is a great deal of evidence that when members of the public form a relationship with a television personality, it can be an intensely personal one. It is a common experience for the television personality to be accosted by members of the public who recognize him and start talking to him as if he knew as much about them as the converse.

EVALUATION OF RESULTS

The potential value of television in changing attitudes and modifying well-established social prejudices – such as the public's attitude to mental illness – was demonstrated in the United Kingdom by the inquiry carried out by the British Broadcasting Corporation into the effects of five television broadcasts in 1957 on 'The Hurt Mind'. It was reported that there had been a small but well-spread increase in the public's acceptance of the principle that mental illness is 'just another illness'; and that the broadcasts were followed by an increase, from 5 per cent (before) to 10 per cent (after), in the proportion of the public aware of mental illness as a major social problem. Essex-Lopresti (646) commented that in Great Britain television is a potentially powerful ally in this field, and that it is disappointing that so few programmes have been devised to turn this to advantage. However, the same author also remarked that various attempts to treat psychiatric subjects in a dramatic way have all failed.

In a personal communication to the Study Group, Fox reported the result of an experiment set up to evaluate the usefulness of television programmes intended to encourage people to apply for immunization; it was found that whereas some 7 or 8 per cent of those who came for immunization did so as a direct result of the programme, in fact the total numbers seeking immunization dropped by one-third. It might be surmised that, whereas the programme had created favourable attitudes in some people, it had increased the sum total of resistance in the community, a finding which, if confirmed on a large scale, would cast considerable doubt on the value of this method of propaganda.

The use of films in public mental health education is now fairly widespread (626, 647). Jacoby (647) has drawn attention to the fact that the usefulness of the film medium in this context is dependent on the presence of personnel qualified to lead a discussion each time a film is shown. An incident was reported to the Study Group in illustration of the danger of not following up the showing of a mental health film with adequate discussion. This particular film gave a highly dramatized portrayal of a woman who had been very strongly attached to her father and later became a successful career woman. When it was shown without opportunity for discussion, it was found that to a considerable number of the viewers it had conveyed the message that the woman's successful career was a consequence of her attachment to her father – which was far from the intention of the film-makers.

Commenting on the use of mass media for mental health

propaganda and education, Ahrenfeldt remarked in a working paper for the Study Group:

'The use of mass media for mental health propaganda and education not only requires the provision of well-organized group discussion, but raises a demand for individual guidance, and for personal advice and help. This is a matter of the greatest importance, which does not appear as yet to have received sufficient attention and thought. Upon the existence of such facilities for guidance and therapeutic "catharsis" will depend the success or failure of this type of education; it is obvious that to arouse interest, concern, and quite possibly in some cases unconscious guilt, without directing such emotional forces into positive, constructive channels, is to run a very serious and unjustifiable risk, at the least of inducing a negative attitude towards mental health, or worse still, the development of over-cautious, over-anxious states of mind and a sense of doubt and uncertainty, in those whom it was proposed to enlighten. It is therefore necessary to ascertain, as Ridenour (632) pointed out, whether it is possible at present to distinguish between arousing concern and arousing anxiety; at what point or in what circumstances concern turns into anxiety; whether the anxiety can be allayed by discussion; what recommendations might be made to discussion leaders, etc.'

The WHO Helsinki conference (635) stressed the serious risk of misinterpretation that attends the use of mass media, which there may be no way of correcting, and the need for far more 'before and after' surveys of public opinion in order to gauge the nature and extent of any change of public attitude, and of any effects contrary to the intention of the educators. The conference also remarked on the danger of building up hypochondriacal or cynical attitudes and unrealistic expectations in the public mind; and the unhelpfulness of stimulating a demand for facilities which cannot be met.

The Study Group were fully cognisant of the fact that all the forms of health education today constitute only a tiny fraction of the tremendous flood of material being introduced by mass media in the course of advertising programmes in most highly developed industrial communities. In some of the less industrialized countries, too, there has recently been an awakening of concern about the possible harmful effects of the mass media – press, television, radio – especially in respect of a feared inundation of the community with commercial advertisements, sex stimulation, violence, and horror. The horror cult has been widely condemned and censured for its pernicious effects, but in fact objective evidence in support of the claim that it does harm is at present not convincing. In a survey made by Himmelweit (421) of the effect of television programmes on children's fears and anxieties, only inconclusive answers were obtained, but it seemed likely that children who were disposed to anxiety might suffer excessively as a result of 'horror'. It is sometimes argued that the presentation of violence and horror on the screen can have a beneficial result in that it enables the vicarious expression of powerful emotions. There is no agreement on this point, although it has been noted, for example, that there is an exceptional record of peace in the community in traditional Balinese society, where there is community-wide involvement in the traditional drama; the drama deals with the more basic emotions, which are given very little expression in normal social life. On the other hand, psychodynamic experience indicates the futility of expecting to work out marked degrees of aggression by vicarious means.

It seems clear that attempts at mental health education through the mass media will be likely to be harmful if the public confuses them with admass techniques, and that they will encounter similar sales resistance if they are seen in this light. We are here on very uncertain ground, because not enough is known in general about the effects of modern propaganda drives in all their various directions, or in particular about the results of the small efforts that are being made to use mass media methods on behalf of mental health education.

THE IMAGE CREATED BY MASS MEDIA

One of the problems that arises in considering the use of the mass media for mental health education is how to control the image that the publicity evokes in the mind of the recipient. A psychiatrist in the Study Group advocated an attempt to create a new kind of image that would help people to understand that there are different degrees of mental health and mental illness, and might also lead to the formation of healthier attitudes to semi-invalidism, unhappiness, and poor human relations.

This idea appears attractive when first considered, partly because progress has undoubtedly been made in evolving propaganda techniques for the creation of new types of images in the public mind. But how such methods could be applied to the complex issues involved in mental health is a more difficult question. There is the additional disadvantage, noted above, of the unfavourable public image that advertisers have, on the whole, created for themselves in their anxiety to sell their wares. Thus, to some extent, the use of mass media techniques (sometimes known as admass) for the creation of new images of mental health should be regarded as the use of a partially devalued currency. As an example of a mishap in the creation of a new image by mass media, a recent experience in Australia may be cited: a major evening newspaper conducts an annual campaign designed to provide firewood and blankets for certain needy old-age pensioners. The campaign has created an erroneous public impression of indigence in old age, whereas the facts show that half of the pensioners are so well off that they do not need to draw their pensions. The social effects of such a misconception might be very considerable.

By far the most common criticism of the mass media in this context, and one that is alleged in many countries, is that they have recourse to sensationalism. We have already reported that supporters of WFMH in the USA have found it difficult to raise money for mental health unless their publicity emphasizes primarily mental illness, hospitals, and the effects of disease. Other countries experience a similar problem, and it is frequently said that in order to get support for a cause one has to show the public an image of the order of a child with a crutch (but never a child looking defective – that is fatal to money-raising hopes). We have discussed elsewhere the dilemma of getting public support for mental hospitals; how to paint a picture of current conditions that is striking enough to elicit a response without frightening off those who need treatment. In France, a recent campaign against alcoholism which underlined the horror aspects, such as harm done to children, has been a relative failure. And in Great Britain, adverse results of propaganda for the prevention of road accidents have led largely to the abandonment of horror methods.

The Study Group was convinced of the need for a higher level of abstract thinking about the role of the mass media for serious propaganda purposes. In countries where the mass media are complex and where numerous diverse agencies, public and private, are advancing their points of view about a variety of good, bad, and indifferent causes, there is a need for some responsible group to concern itself with the overall message that is being conveyed and with the advantages and disadvantages of competing in the same media with commercial advertising. Every fundraising campaign in the medical and social welfare field carries some mental health implications, and programmes on alcoholism, smoking, cancer, and the like tend to benefit or suffer from the effect of parallel campaigns in the field of mental health.

The laudable objectives behind a piece of promotional activity can be nullified by an unforeseen damaging implication. For example, a full-page advertisement carried by a number of American weeklies showed a well-known television figure with his arm round a little boy who was bending down and shading his eyes. The caption was, 'Is your child a sight delinquent?' This was regarded as a piece of good advertising, produced by the National Eye Institute as part of a campaign to encourage the idea that all children's eyes should be examined. However, from the point of view of mental health it carried a most unfortunate message by attaching the word 'delinquent' to children who have defective vision. What the advertisers had intended to convey was 'Are you a delinquent parent in not having had your child's eyes examined?'; but the message that got over to the public was a confused one that included the idea that children who do not see well do badly in school, may truant, and may become delinquent. Although this was a well-meant advertisement, thought out by responsible people in a good cause, it went wrong, and representations had to be made to get it changed.

Another instance of a well-intentioned propaganda effort undertaken by a highly responsible agency was that of a pamphlet produced by the city of Los Angeles with the object of preventing children from getting into motor cars with strangers. Unfortunately, the message that the pamphlet got across to children, generally, was 'A terrible perverted kidnapper may look just like your daddy'.

These examples of projects that failed in their purpose have been selected to illustrate some of the difficulties that are encountered in attempting to promote mental health education through the mass media. Nevertheless, the Study Group concluded that, with due care, these media could be employed with much greater success than they have been hitherto in this area. It must be remembered that, whether or not the mass media are used constructively by mental health educators, they will continue to be used, and often to the disadvantage of mental health, by advertisers and propagandists of all kinds of cause. As remarked earlier, there is a mental health aspect to almost every public campaign aimed at influencing people's thought, whatever the subject.

NEED FOR RESEARCH

What is needed – and this point must be emphasized – is more expert knowledge of the effects of the mass media and of the techniques of applying them, particularly in the field of image creation. Selecting the best agent to undertake mental health education in a particular community is itself a very complex problem; but certain essential criteria may be mentioned. In addition to being an expert in mental health matters, the agent must be well versed in the principles of education, and prepared to work in a team with native-born specialists in educational techniques. Above all, the educators must be acceptable as personalities or as a public image to the people they are seeking to influence, and be placed in a context that is appropriate for the task that they are attempting.

However great the apparent power and influence of the mass media, it is possible that their effectiveness has already been considerably dissipated in many countries by constant over-use, and by the projection of narrow sectional interests and the pursuit of personal profit. In any case it is useless to attempt to influence a whole population over a wide range of mental health issues by means of a single operation employing mass media techniques. Each project must have a particular aim and be specifically directed to meet the needs of a fairly precisely defined body of recipients. In a working paper Ewalt drew attention to the equivocal nature of the information that is presented by studies of the effects on a population of mass education methods for mental health purposes. There is evidence that mass media can change people's attitudes towards mentally ill persons and give them fragmentary knowledge concerning the nature of mental illness, its symptoms and treatment; on the other hand, it appears that people who acquire this knowledge are unable as a rule to recognize these same symptoms or the precursors of illness in themselves or in others. We may add that there is little or no evidence that the mass media have been instrumental in creating or increasing more positive public concepts of mental health.

The task of undertaking mass methods of mental health education falls to different people in different countries. In the Soviet Union the responsibility lies with the Central Institute of Health Education: this body prepares educational materials for those who are carrying out the work – doctors, schoolteachers, and so on – but is not itself regarded as having a direct educational function. This way of doing things tends to create an atmosphere in which mental health workers expect and are expected to be involved in the health education of the public. A similar style of organization is found in Yugoslavia on a provincial basis; in addition, mental health experts actively cooperate with writers, playwrights, and film-makers in producing educational materials on such topics as relationships between children and their parents, attitudes to child-rearing, and so on. A particularly interesting example of a piece of educational material that has resulted from this cooperation is a film which shows how a kitchen appears to a very young child. This is achieved by enlarging the objects in proportion to the child's own body image and by taking shots from his eye level. It is an imaginative approach that deserves application to other aspects of child-rearing.

In the United States, mental health education has been almost exclusively the province of voluntary agencies or private individuals with, in recent years, an increasing tendency for local health authorities to be active in this field. The use of the mass media is still confined to voluntary personnel. In the United Kingdom, France, and a number of other European countries a similar situation prevails but with more direct government action in providing clinical facilities. In these countries the opportunities for promoting government mental health education programmes through the clinics are correspondingly greater. Furthermore, in recent years there have been extensive government campaigns by means of posters and press advertisements on specific burning topics such as cancer, tuberculosis, alcohol and drug addiction, venereal disease, programmes of inoculation, accident prevention, and promotion of milk sales.

To conclude this area of discussion, the Study Group wished to affirm that, given fuller understanding of their potential contribution in this context and the exercise of appropriate safeguards in their application, the mass media – for all their imprecision and the abuses to which they are put – are a valuable and indeed a necessary part of mental health education programmes. To recapitulate briefly: each programme should be treated as an ongoing responsibility with the object of building up a continuing relationship between a particular educator or method and the recipients; for example, by arranging a series of programmes, or by allowing for questions, answers, and some sort of follow-up.

This is especially important in the case of advice columns in newspapers which, if undertaken at all, should be a regular feature of the paper concerned, should deal mainly in general matters in public, and should maintain a system of private correspondence for more specific case problems.

A basic point to be borne in mind is that whereas to the educator the mass media represent a means of disseminating his message to a wide public, to the individual recipient they can have an intensely personal significance: thus the latter may be reading his newspaper in his own home, a paper that he has been taking for twenty years and with which he is strongly identified. With radio and television, the message is projected into the centre of the intimate family group and the personality of the educator becomes to some extent the property of the family; the great disadvantage of these methods is that the educator has no opportunity of joining in the discussion that his programmes provoke, which is perhaps the most valuable part of small group education.

PART FOUR

Bibliography

Bibliography

This bibliography has been compiled with the primary aim of including a significant proportion of the more important and representative publications that have appeared since 1948 in the very wide field of mental health, as well as such other works as have been referred to in the text.

In so vast a field there is necessarily, and fortunately, considerable overlap between subjects and disciplines, which has led to the adoption of a somewhat arbitrary method of classification, for purposes of presentation.

Each section of the bibliography is divided into two parts:

(i) Works identified by individual authors. Here items are arranged alphabetically under authors' names. Works by the same author are given in chronological order, and where there are two or more works by the same author in the same year these are listed alphabetically according to the first letter of the title.

(ii) Works of collective authorship. These publications (reports, studies, etc.) are listed alphabetically under the name of the organization concerned, the title of the work, or the country of origin, as may be appropriate. Where it is necessary, items are given in chronological order or alphabetically by title, as in (i) above.

Abbreviations of titles of periodicals are, in general, those of the *World List of Scientific Periodicals* (3rd edition, London, 1952).

In psychiatry and allied disciplines, the following periodical reviews of the literature will be found to be the most useful:

Monthly – *Excerpta medica, Amsterdam,* Section VIII (Neurology and Psychiatry).

BIBLIOGRAPHY

Annual – *Progress in Neurology and Psychiatry*, Ed. E. A. Spiegel, New York.

Annual –*Year Book of Neurology, Psychiatry and Neurosurgery*, Present Eds. R. P. Mackay, S. B. Wortis & O. Sugar, Chicago.

In other branches of the human sciences concerned, reference should be made to the respective specialized periodicals and yearbooks which periodically review the literature in these fields.

CLASSIFICATION

Preventive Aspects of Mental Health Action

Social and Cross-cultural Aspects of Mental Health Action

Professional Training

Public Education in Mental Health

Additional References

Supplementary Titles

Unnumbered; a selection of more recent works

The Field of Mental Health

MENTAL HEALTH PLANNING AND PERSPECTIVES

1 BROCKINGTON, F. (ed.) 1955. *Mental Health and the World Community*. WFMH, London.

2 DUBOS, R. 1959. *Mirage of Health: Utopias, Progress and Biological Change*. London.

3 KRAPF, E. E. 1959. 'The international approach to the problems of mental health.' *Int. soc. Sci. J.* **11**: 63–71.

4 KRAPF, E. E. 1960. 'The work of the World Health Organization in the field of mental health.' *Ment. Hyg.* **44**: 315–338.

5 KRAPF, E. E. & MOSER, J. 1962. 'Changes of emphasis and accomplishments in mental health work, 1948–1960.' *Ment. Hyg.* **46**: 163–91. (Revised version of a working paper prepared for the Int. Study Group, Roffey Park, June 1961.)

6 LAIGNEL-LAVASTINE, M. & VINCHON, J. 1930. *Les Malades de l'esprit et leurs médecins du XVIe au XIXe siècle*. Paris. P. 14.

7 LEWIS, A. 1958. 'Between guesswork and certainty in psychiatry.' *Lancet* **1**: 171–5, 227–30.

8 PATON, A. C. L. & KIDSON, M. C. (eds.) 1961. *First World Mental Health Year: A Record*. WFMH, London.

9 REES, J. R. 1958. 'The way ahead.' *Amer. J. Psychiat.* **115**: 481–90.

10 SEMELAIGNE, R. 1930. *Les Pionniers de la psychiatrie française*. Tome 1. Paris.

11 THORNTON, E. M. (ed.) 1961. *Planning and Action for Mental Health* (12th & 13th Annual Meetings of WFMH – Barcelona, 1959 & Edinburgh, 1960). WFMH, London.

12 INTERNATIONAL PREPARATORY COMMISSION. 1948. *Mental Health and World Citizenship: A Statement prepared for the International Congress on Mental Health,*

London, 1948. WFMH, London. (English and German texts.)

13 WFMH. 1948. *Third International Congress on Mental Health, London, 1948.* Vol. 1: *History, Development and Organization*; Vol. 2: *Child Psychiatry*; Vol. 3: *Medical Psychotherapy*; Vol. 4: *Mental Hygiene.* 4 vols. WFMH, London.

14 WFMH. 1952. *Proceedings of the Fourth International Congress on Mental Health, Mexico City, 1951.* Mexico, D.F.

15 WFMH. 1954. *Mental Health in Public Affairs: A Report of the Fifth International Congress on Mental Health, Toronto, 1954.* Toronto.

16 WFMH. 1955. *Family Mental Health and the State* (8th Ann. Meeting WFMH, Istanbul, 1955). WFMH, London.

17 WFMH. 1956. *Bericht über die 6. Jahresversammlung der Weltvereinigung für Psychische Hygiene* (6th Ann. Meeting WFMH, Wien, 1953). Wien & Bonn.

18 WFMH. 1956. *Mental Health in Home and School* (9th Ann. Meeting WFMH, Berlin, 1956). WFMH, London.

19 WFMH. 1957. *Growing Up in a Changing World* (10th Ann. Meeting WFMH, Copenhagen, 1957). WFMH, London.

20 WFMH. 1960. *A Brief Record of Eleven Years, 1948–1959, and World Mental Health Year 1960.* WFMH, London.

21 WFMH. 1961. *Mental Health in International Perspective: A Review made in 1961 by an International and Interprofessional Study Group.* WFMH, London.

22 WFMH. 1961. *Proceedings of the VIth International Congress on Mental Health (Paris, 1961). Excerpta med. Int. Congr. Ser.* No. 45. Amsterdam.

23 WHO. 1950. Expert Committee on Mental Health: Report on the 1st Session. *World Hlth Org. tech. Rep. Ser.* 9. Geneva.

24 WHO. 1951. Expert Committee on Mental Health: Report on the 2nd Session. *World Hlth Org. tech. Rep. Ser.* 31. Geneva.

THE CONCEPTUALIZATION OF MENTAL HEALTH

25 COBB, S. 1952. Foreword in *The Biology of Mental Health and Disease*. New York. Pp. xix–xxi.

26 DAVID, H. R. & BRENGELMANN, J. F. (eds.) 1960. *Perspectives in Personality Research*. London.

27 DICKS, H. V. 1959. *Mental Health in the light of Ancient Wisdom*. WFMH, London.

28 EL MAHI, T. 1960. 'Concept of mental health.' *E. Afr. med. J.* **37**: 472–6.

29 ERIKSON, E. H. 1956. 'The problem of ego identity.' *J. Amer. psychoanal. Ass.* **4**: 56–121.

30 GALDSTON, I. (ed.) 1960. *Human Nutrition, Historic and Scientific*. New York.

31 JAHODA, M. 1958. *Current Concepts of Positive Mental Health*. New York.

32 JUNG, C. G. 1958. *The Undiscovered Self* (transl. R. F. C. Hull). London.

33 KRAPF, E. E. 1961. 'The concepts of normality and mental health in psychoanalysis.' *Int. J. Psycho-Anal.* **42**: 439–46.

34 MASSERMAN, J. H. (ed.) 1959. *Individual and Familial Dynamics* (*Science and Psychoanalysis*, Vol. 2). New York. Part II: Familial and Social Dynamics. Pp. 90–214.

35 MASSERMAN, J. H. (ed.) 1960. *Psychoanalysis and Human Values* (*Science and Psychoanalysis*, Vol. 3). New York. Pp. 181–200.

36 MEAD, M. 1959. 'Mental health in world perspective.' In *Culture and Mental Health*, ed. M. K. Opler. New York. Pp. 501–16.

37 MEAD, M. 1962. 'Mental health and the wider world.' *Amer. J. Orthopsychiat.* **32**: 1–4.

38 RÜMKE, H. C. 1954. 'Solved and unsolved problems in mental health.' In *Mental Health in Public Affairs: A Report of the Fifth International Congress on Mental Health*, Toronto. Pp. 157 et seq.

39 SODDY, K. 1950. 'Mental health.' *Int. Hlth Bull. League of Red Cross Societies*, No. 2.

40 SODDY, K. (ed.) 1961. 'Identity.' In *Cross-cultural Studies in Mental Health*. London. Pp. 1–53.
(First published as: *WFMH Introductory Study No. 1*, London, 1957.)

41 SODDY, K. (ed.) 1961. 'Mental health and value systems.' In *Cross-cultural Studies in Mental Health*. London. Pp.55–261.

42 WHEELIS, A. 1958. *The Quest for Identity*. New York.

43 MILBANK MEMORIAL FUND. 1952. *The Biology of Mental Health and Disease* (27th Ann. Conf. Milbank Memorial Fund). New York.

44 PIUS XII. 1960. *Pie XII parle de santé mentale et de psychologie*. Bruxelles.

MENTAL HEALTH AND RELIGION

45 ANDERSON, G. C. 1956. 'Psychiatry's influence on religion.' *Pastoral Psychology*, Sept.

46 ANDERSON, G. C. 1960. *Current Conditions and Trends in Relations between Religion and Mental Health*. New York.

47 APPEL, K. E. *et al.* 1959. 'Religion.' In *American Handbook of Psychiatry*, ed. S. Arieti. New York. Vol. 2: 1777–810.

48 OATES, W. E. 1955. *Religious Factors in Mental Illness*. New York.

49 O'DOHERTY, E. F. 1956. 'Religion and mental health.' *Studies*, Spring. Dublin.

50 TILLICH, P. J. 1960. *The Impact of Psychotherapy on Theological Thought*. New York.
(Also published in *Pastoral Psychology*, Feb. 1960.)

51 ACADEMY OF RELIGION AND MENTAL HEALTH. 1961. *Religion, Culture, and Mental Health* (Proc. 3rd Academy Symposium, Nov. 1959). New York.

PROBLEMS OF COMMUNICATION

52 CAPES, M. & WILSON, A. T. M. (eds.) 1960. *Communication or Conflict – Conferences: Their Nature, Dynamics, and Planning*. London.

53 CUNNINGHAM, J. M. 1952. 'Problems of communication in scientific and professional disciplines.' *Amer. J. Orthopsychiat.* **22**: 445–56.

54 EY, H. 1954. *Etudes psychiatriques.* Paris. Vol. 3: 32–45 (La Classification des maladies mentales).

55 FREMONT-SMITH, F. 1961. 'The interdisciplinary conference.' *Bull. Amer. Inst. biol. Sciences* **11**, No. 11 (Apr.): 17–20 & 32.

56 GLENN, E. S. 1954. 'Semantic difficulties in internationa' communication.' *ETC: A Review of general Semantics* **11**: 163–80.

57 GLENN, E. S. *et al.* 1958. In *ETC: A Review of general Semantics* **15**: 81–151. Special issue on interpretation and intercultural communication (No. 2, Winter 1957–58).

58 RUESCH, J. 1958. 'Communication difficulties among psychiatrists.' In *Integrative Studies (Science and Psychoanalysis,* Vol. 1), ed. J. H. Masserman. New York. Pp. 85–100.

59 STENGEL, E. 1959. 'Classification of mental disorders.' *Bull. World Hlth. Org.* **21**: 601–63.

Clinical Aspects of Mental Health Action

REGIONAL QUESTIONS

60 ARIETI, S. (ed.) 1959. *American Handbook of Psychiatry.* 2 vols. New York.

61 BARTON, W. E. *et al.* 1961. *Impressions of European Psychiatry.* Amer. Psychiatr. Ass., Washington, D.C.

62 BELLAK, L. 1961. *Contemporary European Psychiatry.* New York.

63 CARAVEDO, B. 1959. 'Social psychiatry in Peru.' In *Progress in Psychotherapy*, eds. J. H. Masserman & J. L. Moreno. New York. Vol. 4: 321.

64 CASEY, J. F. & RACKOW, L. L. 1960. *Observations on the Treatment of the Mentally Ill in Europe.* Veterans Admin., Washington, D.C.

65 CHU, L. & LIU, M. 1960. 'Mental diseases in Peking between 1933 and 1943.' *J. ment. Sci.* **106**: 274–80.

66 DAVIES, S. P. 1960. *Toward Community Mental Health: A Review of the First Five Years of Operations under the Community Mental Health Services Act of the State of New York.* New York.

67 DUCHÊNE, H. 1959. *Les Services psychiatriques publics extra-hospitaliers* (Rapport au 57e Congrès de Psychiatrie et de Neurologie de langue française, Tours, 1959). Paris.

68 FIELD, M. G. 1960. 'Approaches to mental illness in Soviet society: some comparisons and conjectures.' *Social Problems* **7**: 277–97.

69 FORSTER, E. F. B. 1962. 'The theory and practice of psychiatry in Ghana.' *Amer. J. Psychother.* **16**: 7–51.

70 KLINE, N. S. 1960. *The Organization of Psychiatric Care and Psychiatric Research in the Union of Soviet Socialist Republics.* New York.

71 KRAPF, E. E. 1959. 'Les troubles mentaux des Africains et les problèmes de la psychiatrie comparée.' *Méd. et Hyg.*, Genève, **17**: 123–30.

72 LAMBO, T. A. 1955. 'The role of cultural factors in paranoid psychosis among the Yoruba tribe (Nigeria).' *J. ment. Sci.* **101**: 239–66.

73 LAMBO, T. A. 1956. 'Neuropsychiatric observations in the Western Region of Nigeria.' *Brit. med. J.* **2**: 1388–94.

74 LAMBO, T. A. 1959. 'Mental health in Nigeria.' *World ment. Hlth.* **11**: 131–8. (Reprinted, ibid., 1961, **13**: 135–41.)

75 LAMBO, T. A. 1960. 'Further neuropsychiatric observations in Nigeria, with comments on the need for epidemiological study in Africa.' *Brit. med. J.* **2**: 1696–704.

76 LAMBO, T. A. 1960. 'The concept and practice of mental health in African cultures.' *E. Afr. med. J.* **37**: 464–71.

77 MARGETTS, E. L. 1960. 'The future for psychiatry in East Africa.' *E. Afr. med. J.* **37**: 448–56.

78 MORA, G. 1959. 'Recent American psychiatric developments.' In *American Handbook of Psychiatry*, ed. S. Arieti. New York. Vol. 1: 20–21.

79 PACHECO E SILVA, A. C. 1960. 'Mental hygiene in underdeveloped countries.' *World ment. Hlth* **12**: 18–23.

80 PATERSON, A. S. 1959. 'The practice of psychiatry in England under the National Health Service, 1948–1959.' *Amer. J. Psychiat.* **116**: 244–50.

81 SIVADON, P. 1958. 'Problèmes de santé mentale en Afrique noire.' *World ment. Hlth* **10**: 106–19.

82 SIVADON, P. 1959. 'Problèmes de santé mentale aux Caraïbes.' *World ment. Hlth* **11**: 122–30.

83 STOLLER, A. 1957. 'An Australian looks at the underdeveloped world.' In *Mental Health and the World Community*, ed. F. Brockington. WFMH, London. Pp. 31–9.

84 STRÖMGREN, E. 1958. 'Mental health service planning in Denmark.' *Danish med. Bull.* **5**: 1–17.

85 TOOTH, G. 1950. *Studies in Mental Illness in the Gold Coast.* Colonial Res. Publ. No. 6. Colonial Office, London.

86 VYNCKE, J. 1957. 'Psychoses et névroses en Afrique centrale.' *Mém. Acad. R. Sci. colon.* Bruxelles, N.S., **5**: fasc. 5.

87 WORTIS, J. 1961. 'A psychiatric study tour of the USSR.' *J. ment. Sci.* **107**: 119–56.

88 CCTA/CSA. 1960. *Mental Disorders and Mental Health in Africa South of the Sahara (Bukavu, 1958)*. Publ. No. 35. London.

89 *East African med. J.*, 1960. **37**: 443–85 (No. 6, June). Special Number: World Mental Health Year, 1960.

90 'The social problem of epilepsy in Peru.' 1960. *Amer. J. Psychiat.* **117**: 163–4.

91 WHO. 1959. *Seminar on Mental Health in Africa South of the Sahara (Brazzaville, 1958): Final Report.* WHO Regional Office for Africa, Brazzaville.

LOCAL PROGRAMMES

92 CARSE, J., PANTON, N. E. & WATT, A. 1958. 'A district mental health service: The Worthing experiment.' *Lancet* **1**: 39–41.

93 COLEMAN, M. D. & ZWERLING, I. 1959. 'The psychiatric emergency clinic: A flexible way of meeting mental health needs.' *Amer. J. Psychiat.* **115**: 980–4.

94 FREEMAN, H. L. 1960. 'Oldham and District psychiatric service.' *Lancet* **1**: 218–21.

95 LEMKAU, P. V. & CROCETTI, G. M. 1961. 'The Amsterdam municipal psychiatric service: A psychiatric-sociological review.' *Amer. J. Psychiat.* **117**: 779–83.

96 LEYBERG, J. T. 1959. 'A district psychiatric service: The Bolton pattern.' *Lancet* **2**: 282–4.

97 LIN, T. 1961. 'Evolution of mental health programmes in Taiwan.' *Amer. J. Psychiat.* **117**: 961–71.

98 QUERIDO, A. 1954. 'Domiciliary psychiatry: The Amsterdam experiment.' *Brit. med. J.* **2**: 1043.

99 QUERIDO, A. 1956. 'Early diagnosis and treatment services.' In *The Elements of a Community Mental Health Program.* Milbank Memorial Fund, New York. Pp. 158–181.

100 EDINBURGH CORPORATION. 1959. *Mental Health Services – Edinburgh: A Plan for Co-ordinated Development*. Report by a Medical Working Party. Edinburgh.

101 NEW YORK STATE. 1954. *New Program for Community Mental Health Services*. Dept. of Mental Hygiene, Albany, N.Y.

102 WHO. 1959. Conference on Mental Hygiene Practice (Helsinki, 1959). Report of Committee B: Community Psychiatric Services. WHO Regional Office for Europe, Copenhagen. (Duplicated document.)

SURVEYS AND EPIDEMIOLOGICAL STUDIES

103 BLACKER, C. P. 1946. *Neurosis and the Mental Health Services*. London.

104 FELIX, R. H. & KRAMER, M. 1953. 'Extent of the problem of mental disorders.' *Ann. Amer. Acad. polit. soc. Sci.* 1953: 5–14.

105 FREMMING, K. H. 1947. *Morbid Risk of Mental Diseases in an Average Danish Population*. Copenhagen.
(Also published as: *The Expectation of Mental Infirmity in a Sample of a Danish Population*. London, 1951.)

106 HALLGREN,B.&SJÖGREN,T. 1959. 'A clinical and genetico-statistical study of schizophrenia and low-grade mental deficiency in a large Swedish rural population.' *Acta psychiat.* **35,** *Suppl.* 140. Copenhagen.

107 HOCH,P.H.&ZUBIN,J. (eds.) 1961. *Comparative Epidemiology of the Mental Disorders* (Proc. 49th Ann. Meeting Amer. Psychopathol. Ass., 1959). New York.

108 HUGHES, C. C. *et al.* 1960. *People of Cove and Woodlot (The Stirling County Study of Psychiatric Disorder and Sociocultural Environment,* Vol. 2). New York.

109 JACO, E. G. 1960. *The Social Epidemiology of Mental Disorders: A Psychiatric Survey of Texas*. New York.

110 KRAMER, M. 1953. 'Long-range studies of mental hospital patients, an important area for research in chronic disease.' *Milbank mem. Fund Quart.* **31**: 253–64.

III KRAMER, M.1957. 'A discussion of the concepts of incidence and prevalence as related to epidemiologic studies of mental disorders.' *Amer. J. publ. Hlth* **47**: 826–40.

112 LEIGHTON, A. H. 1959. *My Name is Legion (The Stirling County Study of Psychiatric Disorder and Sociocultural Environment*, Vol. 1). New York.

113 MURPHY, J. M. 1962. 'Cross-cultural studies of the prevalence of psychiatric disorders.' *World ment. Hlth* **14**: 53–65.

114 NORRIS, V. 1959. *Mental Illness in London* (Maudsley Monogr. No. 6). London.

115 OPLER, M. K. 1958. 'Epidemiological studies of mental illness: methods and scope of the Midtown study in New York.' In *Symposium on Preventive and Social Psychiatry* (April 1957). Walter Reed Army Institute of Research, Washington, D.C. Pp. 111–47.

116 PASAMANICK, B. (ed.) 1959. *Epidemiology of Mental Disorder*. Amer. Ass. Advanc. Sci., Washington, D.C.

117 PASAMANICK, B. 1961. 'Survey of mental disease in urban population: IV. Approach to total prevalence rates.' *Arch. gen. Psychiatr.* **5**: 151–5.

118 PLUNKETT, R. J. & GORDON, J. E. 1960. *Epidemiology and Mental Illness*. New York.

119 PRIMROSE, E. J. R. 1962. *Psychological Illness: A Community Study*. (Re: General practice.) London.

120 REID, D. D. 1960. *Epidemiological Methods in the Study of Mental Disorders* (World Hlth Org. publ. Hlth Papers 2). Geneva.

121 RÜMKE, H. C. 1961. 'Identification of mental disorder and its causes.' In *Planning and Action for Mental Health*, ed. E. M. Thornton. WFMH, London. Pp. 222–8.

122 SHEPHERD, M. 1957. *A Study of the Major Psychoses in an English County* (Maudsley Monogr. No. 3). London.

123 SJÖGREN, T. & LARSSON, T. 1959. 'The changing age-structure in Sweden and its impact on mental illness.' *Bull. World Hlth. Org.* **21**: 569–82.

124 SROLE, L. *et al.* 1962. *Mental Health in the Metropolis* (Midtown Manhattan Study). New York.

125 ZUBIN, J. (ed.) 1961. *Field Studies in the Mental Disorders* (Proc. Work Conf., Amer. Psychopathol. Ass., 1959). New York.

126 GROUP FOR THE ADVANCEMENT OF PSYCHIATRY (GAP). 1961. *Problems of Estimating Changes in Frequency in Mental Disorders.* Report No. 50. New York.

127 JAPAN. 1959. Report of the statistical survey of the mentally disordered in 1954. Ministry of Health & Welfare, Tokyo. (Duplicated document.)

128 MILBANK MEMORIAL FUND. 1950. *Epidemiology of Mental Disorder.* New York.

129 WHO. 1960. Epidemiology of Mental Disorders: 8th Report of the Expert Committee on Mental Health. *World Hlth Org. tech. Rep. Ser.* 185. Geneva.

130 WHO. 1961. 'The epidemiology of mental disorders.' *World Hlth Org. Chron.* **15**: 68.

CLINICAL ACTION IN THE COMMUNITY

131 AHRENFELDT, R. H. 1958. *Psychiatry in the British Army in the Second World War.* London & New York.

132 ibid. 'Practical Considerations on the Disposal of Delinquents in the Army.' Appendix A, pp. 264–8.

133 BIERER, J. 1960. 'Past, present and future.' *Int. J. soc. Psychiat.* **6**: 165–73.

134 BIERER, J. 1961. 'Day hospitals: further developments.' *Int. J. soc. Psychiat.* **7**: 148–51.

135 EHRHARDT, H. *et al.* (eds.) 1958. *Psychiatrie und Gesellschaft: Ergebnisse und Probleme der Sozialpsychiatrie.* Bern & Stuttgart.

136 FERGUSON, R. S. 1961. 'Side-effects of community care.' *Lancet* **1**: 931–2.

137 GINZBERG, E. *et al.* 1959. *The Ineffective Soldier: Lessons for Management and the Nation.* Vol. 1: *The Lost Divisions*;

Vol. 2: *Breakdown and Recovery*; Vol. 3: *Patterns of Performance*. 3 vols. New York.

138 GREENBLATT, M., LEVINSON, D. J. & KLERMAN, G. J. 1961. *Mental Patients in Transition*. Springfield, Ill.

139 HORDER, J. 1961. The Role of Public Health Officers and General Practitioners in Mental Health Care (Working Paper No. 1, May 1961). WHO Expert Committee on Mental Health, Geneva, Oct.–Nov. 1961. (Duplicated document.)

140 JONES, M. 1961. 'Intra and extramural community psychiatry.' *Amer. J. Psychiat.* **117**: 748–7.

141 JONES, M. & RAPOPORT, R. N. 1955. 'Administrative and social psychiatry.' *Lancet* **2**: 386–8.

142 LEIGHTON, A. H., CLAUSEN, J. A. & WILSON, R. N. (eds.) 1957. *Explorations in Social Psychiatry*. New York.

143 MACMILLAN, D. 1958. 'Community treatment of mental illness.' *Lancet* **2**: 201–4.

144 MACMILLAN, D. 1961. 'Community mental health services and the mental hospital.' *World ment. Hlth* **13**: 46–58.

145 MAY, A. R. 1961. 'Prescribing community care for the mentally ill.' *Lancet* **1**: 760–1.

146 MCKERRACHER, D. G. 1961. 'Psychiatric care in transition.' *Ment. Hyg.* **45**: 3–9.

147 REES, T. P. 1957. 'Back to moral treatment and community care.' *J. ment. Sci.* **103**: 303–13.

148 ROLLIN, H. R. 1960. 'Social psychiatry in Britain.' *Trans. Coll. Physicians Philad. Ser. 4*, **27**: 126–37.

149 TITMUSS, R. M. 1961. As reported in *Lancet* **1**: 609.

150 VEIL, C. 1959. 'Introduction à la psychiatrie sociale.' *Bull. Centre Etudes Rech. psychotech.* **8**: 29–38.

151 'Doubtful progress in psychiatry' (Correspondence). 1960. *Lancet* **2**: 261, 371, 433, 599–600.

152 ENGLAND & WALES. 1951. *Report of the Committee on Social Workers in the Mental Health Services*. Ministry of Health, London.

153 WHO. 1954. *European Seminar on Mental Health Aspects of*

Public Health Practice (Amsterdam, 1953). WHO Regional Office for Europe, Geneva.

154 WHO. 1955. 'Mental health through public health practice.' *World Hlth Org. Chron.* **9**: 247–53.

155 WHO. 1959. Social Psychiatry and Community Attitudes: 7th Report of the Expert Committee on Mental Health. *World Hlth Org. tech. Rep. Ser.* 177. Geneva.

THE PSYCHIATRIC HOSPITAL

I. *Changing Patterns of Organization*

156 BAKER, A. A. 1958. 'Breaking up the mental hospital.' *Lancet* **2**: 253–5.

157 BAKER, A. A., DAVIES, R. L. & SIVADON, P. 1959. *Psychiatric Services and Architecture.* (World Hlth Org. publ. Hlth Papers 1). Geneva.

158 BARR, A., GOLDING, D. & PARNELL, R. W. 1962. 'Recent critical trends in mental hospital admissions in the Oxford Region.' *J. ment Sci.* **108**: 59–67.

159 BARTON, R., ELKES, A. & GLEN, F. 1961. 'Unrestricted visiting in a mental hospital: An inquiry into its effects and nursing-staff attitudes.' *Lancet* **1**: 1220–2.

160 BATEMAN, J. F. 1949. In *Better Care in Mental Hospitals* (Proc. 1st Mental Hospital Institute, Amer. Psychiat. Ass.). Washington, D.C. Appendix III, p. 187.

161 BERESFORD, C. 1959. Annual Report of The Retreat mental hospital, York, for 1959 – as quoted in *Lancet* **2**: 680.

162 BRIDGMAN, R. F. 1955. *The Rural Hospital: Its Structure and Organization* (World Hlth Org. Monogr. Ser. 21). Geneva.

163 CLARK, D. H. 1958. 'Administrative therapy: Its clinical importance in the mental hospital.' *Lancet* **1**: 805–8.

164 COOPER, A. B. & EARLY, D. F. 1961. 'Evolution in the mental hospital: Review of a hospital population.' *Brit. med. J.* **1**: 1600–3.

165 FLECK, S. *et al.* 1957. 'Interaction between hospital staff and families.' *Psychiatry* **20**: 343–50.

166 GARRATT, F. N., LOWE, C. R. & MCKEOWN, T. 1958. 'Institutional care of the mentally ill.' *Lancet* 1: 682–4.

167 GREENBLATT, M. *et al.* 1955. *From Custodial to Therapeutic Patient Care in Mental Hospitals.* New York. (Cf. 'Relation of the hospital to the community.' Pp. 212–34.)

168 HARPER, J. 1959. 'Out-patient adult psychiatric clinics.' *Brit. med. J.* 1: 357–60.

169 JONES, K. & SIDEBOTHAM, R. 1962. *Mental Hospitals at Work.* London.

170 KINGSTON, F. E. 1962. 'Trends in mental-hospital population and their effect on planning.' *Lancet* 2: 49.

171 LINDSAY, J. S. B. 1962. 'Trends in mental-hospital population and their effect on planning.' *Lancet* 1: 1354–5.

172 MACMILLAN, D. 1958. 'Hospital-community relationships.' In *An Approach to the Prevention of Disability from Chronic Psychoses: The Open Mental Hospital within the Community.* Milbank Memorial Fund, New York. Pp. 29–50.

173 MAIN, T. F. 1958. 'Mothers with children in a psychiatric hospital.' *Lancet* 2: 845–7.

174 NORTON, A. 1961. 'Mental hospital ins and outs: A survey of patients admitted to a mental hospital in the past 30 years.' *Brit. med. J.* 1: 528–36.

175 OVERHOLSER, W. 1955. 'The present status of the problems of release of patients from mental hospitals.' *Psychiat. Quart.* 29: 372–80.

176 REPOND, A. 1960. 'Santé mentale et hôpital psychiatrique.' *Rev. Méd. prév.* 5: 276–98.

177 RICHTER, D. (ed.) 1950. *Perspectives in Neuropsychiatry.* London.

178 SANDS, S. L. 1959. 'Discharges from mental hospitals.' *Amer. J. Psychiat.* 115: 748–50.

179 SHAW, D. & SAMUEL, A. 1959. 'Medical administration in psychiatric hospitals.' *Lancet* 2: 170–2.

180 SIVADON, P. 1959. 'Transformation d'un service d'aliénés

de type classique en un centre de traitement actif et de ré-adaptation sociale.' *Bull. World Hlth Org.* **21**: 593–600.

181 SMITH, S. *et al.* 1960. 'Metamorphosis of a mental hospital.' *Lancet* **2**: 592–3.

182 TOOTH, G. C. 1958. 'The psychiatric hospital and its place in a mental health service.' *Bull. World Hlth Org.* **19**: 363–87.

183 TOOTH, G. C. & BROOKE, E.M. 1961. 'Trends in the mental hospital population and their effect on future planning.' *Lancet* **1**: 710–13.

184 'A different hospital.' 1959. *Lancet* **2**: 221–2.

185 'A look at mental hospitals.' 1962. *Lancet* **1**: 900.

186 ENGLAND & WALES. 1962. *A Hospital Plan for England and Wales.* London.
(Preface and general review reprinted verbatim in *Brit. med. J.* 1962, **1**: 244–51.)

187 'Gains in outpatient psychiatric services, 1959.' 1960. *Publ. Hlth Rep.* **75**: 1092–4. Washington, D.C.

188 'Hospital services for the mentally ill.' 1961. *Brit. med. J.* **1**: 1184.

II. *The Therapeutic Community*

189 CAUDILL, W. 1958. *The Psychiatric Hospital as a Small Society.* Cambridge, Mass.

190 CROCKET, R. W. 1960. 'Doctors, administrators, and therapeutic communities.' *Lancet* **2**: 359–63.

191 JONES, M. *et al.* 1952. *Social Psychiatry: A Study of Therapeutic Communities.* London.

192 MAIN, T. F. 1946. 'The hospital as a therapeutic institution.' *Bull. Menninger Clin.* **10**: 66–70.

193 STANTON, A. H. & SCHWARTZ, M. S. 1954. *The Mental Hospital: A Study of Institutional Participation in Psychiatric Illness and Treatment.* New York.

194 WALTER REED ARMY INSTITUTE OF RESEARCH. 1958. 'Panel on the development of a therapeutic milieu in the mental hospital.' In *Symposium on Preventive and Social Psychiatry (April 1957).* Washington, D.C. Pp. 455–529.

195 WHO. 1953. Expert Committee on Mental Health: 3rd Report. *World Hlth Org. tech. Rep. Ser.* 73. Geneva.

III. *Day and Night Hospitals*

196 BIERER, J. 1951. *The Day Hospital: An Experiment in Social Psychiatry and Syntho-Analytic Psychotherapy.* London.

197 BIERER, J. 1959. 'Theory and practice of psychiatric day hospitals.' *Lancet* 2: 901–2.

198 BIERER, J. & BROWNE, I. W. 1960. 'An experiment with a psychiatric night hospital.' *Proc. R. Soc. Med.* 53: 930–2.

199 BOAG, T. J. 1960. 'Further developments in the day hospital.' *Amer. J. Psychiat.* 116: 801–6.

200 CAMERON, D. E. 1956. 'The day hospital.' In *The Practice of Psychiatry in General Hospitals* by A. E. Bennett *et al.* Berkeley & Los Angeles, Calif. Pp. 134–50.

201 CRAFT, M. 1959. 'Psychiatric day hospitals.' *Amer. J. Psychiat.* 116: 251–4.

202 FARNDALE, J. 1961. *The Day Hospital Movement in Great Britain.* Oxford.

203 FOX, R. *et al.* 1960. 'Psychiatric day hospitals.' *Lancet* 1: 824–5.

204 FREEMAN, H. L. 1960. 'The day hospital.' *World ment. Hlth* 12: 192–8.

205 GOSHEN, G. E. 1959. 'New concepts of psychiatric care with special reference to the day hospital.' *Amer. J. Psychiat.* 115: 808–11.

IV. *Rehabilitation*

206 BRIDGER, H. 1946. 'The Northfield experiment.' *Bull. Menninger Clin.* 10: 71–6.

207 GRAYSON, M. *et al.* 1952. *Psychiatric Aspects of Rehabilitation.* New York Univ., Bellevue Med. Center, New York.

208 GREENBLATT, M. & SIMON, B. (eds.) 1959. *Rehabilitation of the Mentally Ill.* Amer. Ass. Advanc. Sci., Washington, D.C.

209 LE GUILLANT, L. *et al.* 1958. 'Une réforme de l'assistance psychiatrique: Le service médico-social de secteur.' *Tech. hosp.* **14**: 34.

210 WHO. 1958. Expert Committee on Medical Rehabilitation: 1st Report. *World Hlth Org. tech. Rep. Ser.* 158. Geneva.

PSYCHOTHERAPY

211 FERENCZI, S. 1955. *Final Contributions to the Problems and Methods of Psycho-Analysis* (ed. M. Balint). London. P. 141.

212 FROMM-REICHMANN, F. & MORENO, J. L. (eds.) (Vol. 1); MASSERMAN, J. H. & MORENO, J. L. (eds.) (Vols. 2–5). 1956–60. *Progress in Psychotherapy.* 5 vols. New York.

213 MASSERMAN, J. H. & MORENO, J. L. (eds.) 1959. *Progress in Psychotherapy*, Vol 4: *Social Psychotherapy.* New York.

PHARMACOTHERAPY

214 BRILL, H. & PATTON, R. E. 1959. 'Analysis of population reduction in New York State mental hospitals during the first four years of large scale therapy with psychotropic drugs.' *Amer. J. Psychiat.* **116**: 495–509.

215 GARATTINI, S. & GHETTI, V. (eds.) 1957. *Psychotropic Drugs* (Proc. Int. Symposium on Psychotropic Drugs, Milan 1957). Amsterdam.

216 GELBER, I. 1959. *Release Mental Patients on Tranquillizing Drugs and the Public Health Nurse.* New York.

217 GROSS, M. 1960. 'The impact of ataractic drugs on a mental hospital out-patient clinic.' *Amer. J. Psychiat.* **117**, 444–7.

218 GUPTA, J. C., DEB, A. K. & KAHALI, B. S. 1943. 'Preliminary observations on the use of *Rauwolfia serpentina* Benth. in the treatment of mental disorders.' *Indian med. Gaz.* **78**: 547–9.

219 HOCH, P. H. 1959. 'Drug therapy.' In *American Handbook of Psychiatry*, ed. S. Arieti. New York. Vol. 2: 1541–51.

220 HUTCHINSON, J. T. & SMEDBERG, D. 1960. 'Phenelzine ("Nardil") in the treatment of endogenous depression.' *J. ment. Sci.* **106**: 704–10.

221 HUTCHINSON, R. 1953. 'Modern treatment.' *Brit. med J.* **1**: 671.

222 JACOBSEN, E. 1959. 'The comparative pharmacology of some psychotropic drugs.' *Bull. World Hlth Org.* **21**: 411–93.

223 KILOH, L. G. & BALL, J. R. B. 1961. 'Depression treated with imipramine ("Tofranil"): A follow-up study.' *Brit. med. J.* **1**: 168–71.

224 KLINE, N. S. 1959. 'Psychopharmaceuticals: Effects and side-effects.' *Bull. World Hlth Org.* **21**: 397–410.

225 KLINE, N. S. (ed.) 1959. *Psychopharmacology Frontiers* (2nd Int. Congr. Psychiatry: Proc. Psychopharmacol. Symposium). Boston.

226 LINDEMANN, E. 1959. 'The relation of drug-induced mental changes to psychoanalytical theory.' *Bull. World Hlth Org.* **21**: 517–26.

227 LINN, E. L. 1959. 'Sources of uncertainty in studies of drugs affecting mood, mentation or activity.' *Amer. J. Psychiat.* **116**: 97–103.

228 PRINCE, R. 1960. 'The use of *Rauwolfia* for the treatment of psychoses by Nigerian native doctors.' *Amer. J. Psychiat.* **117**: 147–9.

229 REES, L., BROWN, A. C. & BENAIM, S. 1961. 'A controlled trial of imipramine ("Tofranil") in the treatment of severe depressive states.' *J. ment. Sci.* **107**: 552–9.

230 REES, L. & DAVIES, B. 1961. 'A controlled trial of phenelzine ("Nardil") in the treatment of severe depressive illness.' *J. ment. Sci.* **107**: 560–6.

231 SANDISON, R. A. 1959. 'The role of psychotropic drugs in group therapy.' *Bull. World Hlth Org.* **21**: 505–15.

232 SANDISON, R. A. 1959. 'The role of psychotropic drugs in individual therapy.' *Bull. World Hlth Org.* **21**: 495–503.

233 UHR, L. & MILLER, J. G. (eds.) 1960. *Drugs and Behavior.* New York.

234 WATT, J. M. & BREYER-BRANDWIJK, M. G. 1962. *The Medicinal and Poisonous Plants of Southern and Eastern Africa.* (2nd ed.) Edinburgh. Pp. 95–100.

235 PIUS XII. 1960. 'Psychiatrie et psychopharmacologie (1958).' In *Pie XII parle de santé mentale et de psychologie.* Bruxelles. Pp. 72–75 (and cf. E. E. Krapf, Préface, p. 10).

236 WHO. 1958. Ataractic and Hallucinogenic Drugs in Psychiatry; Report of a Study Group. *World Hlth Org. tech. Rep. Ser.* 152. Geneva.

PSYCHIATRY IN THE GENERAL HOSPITAL

237 BENNETT, E. A. *et al.* 1956. *The Practice of Psychiatry in General Hospitals.* Berkeley & Los Angeles, Calif.

238 BENNETT, A. E. 1959. 'Problems in establishing and maintaining psychiatric units in general hospitals.' *Amer. J. Psychiat.* 115: 974–9.

239 BROOK, C. P. B. & STAFFORD-CLARK, D. 1961. 'Psychiatric treatment in general wards.' *Lancet* 1: 1159–62.

240 COHEN, N. A. & HALDANE, F. P. 1962. 'Inpatient psychiatry in general hospitals.' *Lancet* 1: 1113–14.

241 COTTON, J. M. 1961. 'The function of a psychiatric service in a general hospital.' *Mental Hosp.*, Sept., pp. 4–7.

242 HOENIG, J. & CROTTY, I. M. 1959. 'Psychiatric inpatients in general hospitals.' *Lancet* 2: 122–3.

243 LINN, L. 1955. *A Handbook of Hospital Psychiatry: A Practical Guide to Therapy.* New York.

244 LINN, L. (ed.) 1961. *Frontiers in General Hospital Psychiatry.* New York.

245 MOROSS, H. 1954. 'The administration of a psychiatric service in a general hospital.' *S. Afr. med. J.* 28: 886–9.

246 NOBLE, H. N. 1961. As reported in *Brit. med. J.* 1: 664–5.

247 SMITH, S. 1961. 'Psychiatry in general hospitals: Manchester's integrated scheme.' *Lancet* 1: 1158–9.

248 'Psychiatry in the general hospital.' 1962. *Lancet* 1: 1107.

PSYCHIATRY IN OBSTETRIC PRACTICE

249 HARGREAVES, G. R. 1955. 'Obstetrics and psychiatry.'
Lancet 1: 39–40.
250 MORRIS, N. 1960. 'Human relations in obstetric practice.'
Lancet 1: 913–15.
251 ENGLAND & WALES. 1961. Human Relations in Obstetrics.
Ministry of Health, London.

PSYCHIATRY IN GENERAL PRACTICE

252 BALINT, M. 1957. The Doctor, his Patient and the Illness.
London.
253 FRANKLIN, L. M. 1960. 'An appraisal of psychiatry in
general practice.' Brit. med. J. 2: 451–3.
254 KRAPF, E. E. 1956. 'Tâches et possibilités du médecin de
famille dans le domaine de l'hygiène mentale.' Arch.
suisses Neurol. Psychiat. 77: 47–56.
(English transl.: 'The family doctor's tasks and opportunities in the field of mental hygiene.' J. Amer. med.
Women's Ass., 1957, 12: 212-15.)
255 LEMERE, F. & KRAABEL, A. B. 1959. 'The general practitioner and the psychiatrist.' Amer. J. Psychiat. 116: 518–
521.
256 WATTS, C. A. H. 1958. 'Management of chronic psycho-
neurosis in general practice.' Lancet 2: 362–4.
257 COLLEGE OF GENERAL PRACTITIONERS. 1958. 'Psychological medicine in general practice.' Brit. med. J. 2:
585–90.

THE MENTAL HEALTH OF THE GENERAL HOSPITAL

258 BARNES, E. 1959. 'Mental health in general hospitals.'
World ment. Hlth 11: 43–7.
259 BARNES, E. 1961. People in Hospital. London.
260 BLUESTONE, E. M. 1958. 'Fear in hospital practice: Some
advantages of home care.' Lancet 1: 1083–4.
261 HEASMAN, G. A. 1962. 'The patient, the doctor and the
hospital.' Lancet 2: 59–62.

262 STATHAM, C. 1959. 'Noise and the patient in hospital: A personal investigation.' *Brit. med. J.* **2**: 1247–8.

263 ENGLAND & WALES. 1953. *The Reception and Welfare of In-Patients in Hospitals.* Ministry of Health, London.

264 ENGLAND & WALES. 1961. *The Pattern of the In-Patient's Day.* Ministry of Health, London.

265 KING EDWARD'S HOSPITAL FUND FOR LONDON. 1958. *Noise Control in Hospitals.* London. (Cf. *Lancet*, 1958, **2**: 1269.)

266 KING EDWARD'S HOSPITAL FUND FOR LONDON. 1962. *Information Booklets for Patients.* London. (Cf. *Lancet*, 1962, **1**: 1392–3.)

267 SCOTTISH ASS. MENTAL HEALTH. 1960. *Report of Scottish Study Group on Psychological Problems in General Hospitals.* Edinburgh.

THE MENTAL HEALTH OF CHILDREN

I. *Clinical Problems*

268 BRADLEY, C. 1941. *Schizophrenia in Childhood.* New York. Pp. 21–4.

269 BROCK, J. F. & AUTRET, M. 1952. *Kwashiorkor in Africa* (World Hlth Org. Monogr. Ser. 8). Geneva.

270 FREEDMAN, A. M. 1959. 'Day hospitals for severely schizophrenic children.' *Amer. J. Psychiat.* **115**: 893–8.

271 GEBER, M. & DEAN, R. F. A. 1955. 'Psychological factors in the aetiology of kwashiorkor.' *Bull. World Hlth Org.* **12**: 471–5.

272 JELLIFFE, D. B. 1955. *Infant Nutrition in the Subtropics and Tropics* (World Hlth Org. Monogr. Ser. 29). Geneva.

273 KANNER, L. 1959. 'Trends in child psychiatry.' *J. ment. Sci.* **105**: 581–93.

274 LORAND, S. & SCHNEER, H. I. (eds.) 1961. *Adolescents: Psychoanalytic Approach to Problems and Therapy.* New York.

275 LURIA, A. K. 1961. *The Role of Speech in the Regulation of Normal and Abnormal Behaviour* (ed. J. Tizard). Oxford.

276 MOSSE, H. L. 1958. 'The misuse of the diagnosis, childhood schizophrenia.' *Amer. J. Psychiat.* **114**: 791–4.

277 SHAGASS, C. & PASAMANICK, B. (eds.) 1960. *Child Development and Child Psychiatry*. In Tribute to Dr Arnold Gesell in his Eightieth Year. Washington, D.C.

278 SODDY, K. 1960. *Clinical Child Psychiatry*. London.

279 TANNER, J. M. & INHELDER, B. (eds.) 1956–60. *Discussions on Child Development*. 4 vols. London.

280 TIZARD, J. P. M. *et al.* 1959. 'The role of the paediatrician in mental illness.' *Lancet* **2**: 193–5.

281 AMERICAN PSYCHIATRIC ASSOCIATION. 1957. *Psychiatric Inpatient Treatment of Children*. Washington, D.C.

282 CENTRE INTERNATIONAL DE L'ENFANCE. 1953. *Les Problèmes de l'enfance dans les pays tropicaux de l'Afrique* (Brazzaville, 1952). Paris. Pp. 315–61.

II. *Organization of Services*

283 BUCKLE, D. & LEBOVICI, S. 1960. *Child Guidance Centres* (World Hlth Org. Monogr. Ser. 40). Geneva.

284 CONNELL, P. H. 1961. 'The day hospital approach in child psychiatry.' *J. ment. Sci.* **107**: 969–77.

285 CREAK, M. 1959. 'Child health and child psychiatry: neighbours or colleagues?' *Lancet* **1**: 481–5.

286 POLLAK, O. *et al.* 1952. *Social Science and Psychotherapy for Children*. New York.

287 SMALLPEICE, V. 1958. 'Children as day patients.' *Lancet* **2**: 1366–7.

288 ENGLAND & WALES. 1955. *Report of the Committee on Maladjusted Children*. Ministry of Education, London.

289 WHO. 1952. *Scandinavian Seminar on Child Psychiatry and Child Guidance Work* (Lillehammer, 1952). WHO Regional Office for Europe, Geneva.

290 WHO. 1952. Joint Expert Committee on the Physically Handicapped Child: 1st Report. *World Hlth Org. tech. Rep. Ser.* 58. Geneva.

III. *Children in Hospital*

291 CAPES, M. 1955. 'The child in hospital.' *Bull. World Hlth Org.* 12: 427–70.

292 ILLINGWORTH, R. S. 1958. 'Children in hospital.' *Lancet* 2: 165–71.

293 TREADGOLD, S. 1960. 'Billy goes to hospital.' *Med. biol. Illustr.* 10: 191–6.

294 BRITISH PAEDIATRIC ASS. 1959. 'The welfare of children in hospital.' *Brit. med. J.* 1: 166–9.

295 ENGLAND & WALES. 1959. *The Welfare of Children in Hospital.* Ministry of Health, London.

SOME SPECIFIC AREAS OF MENTAL HEALTH CONCERN

I. *Addiction*

296 DUHL, L. J. 1959. 'Alcoholism: The public health approach – A new look from the viewpoint of human ecology.' *Quart. J. Stud. Alc.* 20: 112–25.

297 JELLINEK, E. M. 1960. *The Disease Concept of Alcoholism.* New Haven.

298 JELLINEK, E. M. *et al.* 1955. 'The "craving" for alcohol: A symposium by members of the WHO Expert Committees on Mental Health and on Alcohol.' *Quart J. Stud. Alc.* 16: 34–66.

299 KILOH, L. G. & BRANDON, S. 1962. 'Habituation and addiction to amphetamines.' *Brit. med. J.* 2: 40–3.

300 KRUSE, H. D. (ed.) 1961. *Alcoholism as a Medical Problem.* New York.

301 CALIFORNIA. 1961. *Reports of the Division of Alcoholic Rehabilitation of the Department of Public Health (State of California).* Publ. No. 1: A Study of Community Concepts and Definitions (Pt. I); Publ. No. 2: Selected Aspects of the Prospective Follow-up Study (a preliminary review); Publ. No. 3: Criminal Offenders and Drinking Involvement (a preliminary analysis).

302 WHO. 1951. *European Seminar and Lecture Course on Alcoholism* (Copenhagen, 1951). WHO Regional Office for Europe, Geneva.

303 WHO. 1951–55. Expert Committee on Mental Health – Alcoholism Sub-committee: 1st and 2nd Reports; Expert Committee on Alcohol: 1st Report; Alcohol and Alcoholism: Report of an Expert Committee. *World Hlth Org. tech. Rep. Ser.* 42, 48, 84, 94. Geneva.

304 WHO. 1955. *European Seminar on the Prevention and Treatment of Alcoholism*: Selected Lectures (Noordwijk, 1954). WHO Regional Office for Europe, Geneva. (Reprinted from *Quart. J. Stud. Alc.* 1954, **15**, and 1955, **16**.)

305 WHO. 1957–61. Treatment and Care of Drug Addicts: Report of a Study Group; Expert Committee on Addiction-Producing Drugs: 10th and 11th Reports. *World Hlth Org. tech. Rep. Ser.* 131, 188, 211. Geneva.

II. *Ageing*

306 ANDERSON, J. E. (ed.) 1956. *Psychological Aspects of Aging.* Amer. Psychol. Ass., Washington, D.C.

307 BASH, K. W. 1959. 'Mental health problems of aging and the aged from the viewpoint of analytical psychology.' *Bull. World Hlth Org.* **21**: 563–8.

308 COSIN, L. Z. 1955. 'The place of the day hospital in the geriatric unit.' *Int. J. soc. Psychiat.* **1**: No. 2, 33–41.

309 HARGREAVES, G. R. *et al.* 1962. 'Psychiatric and geriatric beds' (Central Consultants and Specialists Committee). As reported in *Brit. med. J.*, *Suppl.* **1**: 209–10.

310 HOCH, P. H. & ZUBIN, J. (eds.) 1961. *Psychopathology of Aging* (Proc. 50th Ann. Meeting Amer. Psychopathol. Ass., 1960). New York.

311 ROTH, M. 1959. 'Mental health problems of aging and the aged.' *Bull. World Hlth Org.* **21**: 527–61, 563–91.

312 SHELDON, J. H. 1960. 'Problems of an ageing population.' *Brit. med. J.* **1**: 1223–30.

313 WHO. 1959. Mental Health Problems of Aging and the Aged: 6th Report of the Expert Committee on Mental Health. *World Hlth Org. tech. Rep. Ser.* 171. Geneva.

III. *Cyclothymia*

314 GIBSON, R. W. *et al.* 1959. 'On the dynamics of the manic-depressive personality.' *Amer. J. Psychiat.* 115: 1101–7.
315 STENSTEDT, A. 1959. 'Involutional melancholia: An etiologic, clinical and social study of endogenous depression in later life, with special reference to genetic factors.' *Acta psychiat.* 34, *Suppl.* 127, Copenhagen.

IV. *Delinquency and Criminality*

316 BOVET, L. 1951. *Psychiatric Aspects of Juvenile Delinquency* (World Hlth Org. Monogr. Ser. 1). Geneva.
317 EDELSTON, H. 1952. *The Earliest Stages of Delinquency: A Clinical Study from the Child Guidance Clinic.* Edinburgh.
318 GIBBENS, T. C. N. 1961. *Trends in Juvenile Delinquency* (World Hlth Org. publ. Hlth Papers 5). Geneva.
319 GITTINS, J. 1952. *Approved School Boys: An Account of the Observation, Classification and Treatment of Boys who come to Aycliffe School.* Home Office, London. (Cf. esp. Pt. III, pp. 84 ff., on psychiatric and psychometric investigations.)
320 JONES, H. 1960. *Reluctant Rebels: Re-education and Group Process in a Residential Community.* London.
321 MANNHEIM, H. & WILKINS, L. T. 1955. *Prediction Methods in Relation to Borstal Training.* London.

V. *Migration*

322 EITINGER, L. 1960. 'The symptomatology of mental disease among refugees in Norway.' *J. ment. Sci.* 106: 947–66.
323 LISTWAN, I. A. 1959. 'Mental disorders in migrants: Further study.' *Med. J. Australia,* April. (Reprinted in *World ment. Hlth,* 1960, 12: 38–45.)

324 MEZEY, A. G. 1960. 'Personal background, emigration and mental disorder in Hungarian refugees.' *J. ment. Sci.* **106**: 618–27.

325 MEZEY, A. G. 1960. 'Psychiatric aspects of human migrations.' *Int. J. soc. Psychiat.* **5**: 245–60.

326 MEZEY, A. G. 1960. 'Psychiatric illness in Hungarian refugees.' *J. ment Sci.* **106**: 628–37.

VI. *Neurosis, and Physical and Psychosomatic Illness*

327 BARKER, R. G. *et al.* 1953. *Adjustment to Physical Handicap and Illness: A Survey of the Social Psychology of Physique and Disability.* Social Sci. Res. Council, New York.

328 BARTON, R. 1959. *Institutional Neurosis.* Bristol.

329 CLECKLEY, H. M. 1959. 'Psychopathic states.' In *American Handbook of Psychiatry*, ed. S. Arieti. New York. Vol. 1: 567–88.

330 COHEN OF BIRKENHEAD, LORD. 1958. 'Epilepsy as a social problem.' *Brit. med. J.* **1**: 672–5.

331 DERNER, G. F. 1953. *Aspects of the Psychology of the Tuberculous.* New York.

332 KRAPF, E. E. 1957. 'On the pathogenesis of epileptic and hysterical seizures.' *Bull. World Hlth Org.* **16**: 749–62.

333 LJUNGBERG, L. 1957. 'Hysteria: A clinical, prognostic and genetic study.' *Acta psychiat.* **32,** *Suppl.* 112. Copenhagen.

334 LOWINGER, P. 1959. 'Leprosy and psychosis.' *Amer. J. Psychiat.* **116**: 32–7.

335 MANSON-BAHR, P. E. C. 1960. 'The physical background of mental disorder in Africans.' *E. Afr. med. J.* **37**: 477–9.

336 MARS, L. 1955. *La Crise de possession: Essais de psychiatrie comparée.* Port-au-Prince, Haiti.

337 MILLER, H. 1961. 'Accident neurosis.' *Brit. med. J.* **1**: 919–25, 992–8.

338 TANNER, J. M. (ed.) 1960. *Stress and Psychiatric Disorder* (2nd. Oxford Conf. Ment. Health Res. Fund). Oxford.

339 WITTKOWER, E. D. 1955. *A Psychiatrist Looks at Tuberculosis.* (2nd ed.) London.

340 WITTKOWER, E. D. & CLEGHORN, R. A. (eds.) 1954. *Recent Developments in Psychosomatic Medicine.* London.

341 WITTKOWER, E. D. & RUSSELL, B. 1953. *Emotional Factors in Skin Disease.* New York.

342 YAP, P. M. 1960. 'The possession syndrome: A comparison of Hong Kong and French findings.' *J. ment. Sci.* **106**: 114-37.

343 ENGLAND & WALES. 1956. *Report of the Sub-committee on the Medical Care of Epileptics.* Ministry of Health, London.

344 PIUS XII. 1960. 'Ressources psycho-spirituelles dans la réhabilitation des malades de la lèpre (1956).' In *Pie XII parle de santé mentale et de psychologie.* Bruxelles. Pp. 68-9.

345 WHO. 1957. Juvenile Epilepsy: Report of a Study Group *World Hlth Org. tech. Rep. Ser.* **130**. Geneva.

346 WHO. 1961. 'Rehabilitation in leprosy.' *World Hlth Org. Chron.* **15**: 111.

VII. *Schizophrenia*

347 BROWN, G. W. 1960. 'Length of stay and schizophrenia: A review of statistical studies.' *Acta psychiat.* **35**: 414-30.

348 FLECK, S. 1960. 'Family dynamics and origin of schizophrenia.' *Psychosom. Med.* **22**: 333-44.

349 LIDZ, T. & FLECK, S. 1959. 'Schizophrenia, human integration, and the role of the family.' In *Etiology of Schizophrenia,* ed. D. Jackson. New York. Pp. 323-45.

350 LIDZ, T. *et al.* 1957. 'The intrafamilial environment of the schizophrenic patient: I. The father.' *Psychiatry* **20**: 329-42.

351 WING, J. K. 1960. 'Pilot experiment in the rehabilitation of long-hospitalized male schizophrenic patients.' *Brit. J. prev. soc. Med.* **14**: 173-80.

352 WING, J. K. & BROWN, G. W. 1961. 'Social treatment of chronic schizophrenia: A constructive survey of three mental hospitals.' *J. ment. Sci.* **107**: 847-61.

353 *Second International Congress for Psychiatry (Zürich).* 1957. *Congress Report.* Zürich. Vol. I (contains a number of papers on schizophrenia in various cultures).

354 WHO. 1959. Report of World Health Organization Study Group on Schizophrenia – Geneva, 9–14 September 1959. *Amer. J. Psychiat.* 115: 865–72.

VIII. *Subnormality*

355 ADAMS, M. (ed.) 1960. *The Mentally Subnormal: The Social Casework Approach.* London.

356 CLARKE, A. M. & CLARKE, A. D. B. (eds.) 1958. *Mental Deficiency: The Changing Outlook.* London.

357 CRAFT, M. 1959. 'Personality disorder and dullness.' *Lancet* I: 856–8.

358 EARL, C. J. C. 1961. *Subnormal Personalities: Their Clinical Investigation and Assessment;* with additional material by H. C. Gunzburg. London.

359 JERVIS, G. A. 1959. 'The mental deficiencies.' In *American Handbook of Psychiatry,* ed. S. Arieti. New York. Vol. 2: 1312–13.

360 LEWIS, A. J. 1960. 'The study of defect' (Adolf Meyer Research Lecture). *Amer. J. Psychiat.* 117: 289–305.

361 O'GORMAN, G. 1958. 'A hospital for the psychotic-defective child.' *Lancet* 2: 951–3.

362 SLAUGHTER, S. S. 1960. *The Mentally Retarded Child and his Parent.* New York.

363 TIZARD, J. 1953. 'The prevalence of mental subnormality.' *Bull. World Hlth Org.* 9: 423–40.

364 TIZARD, J. & GRAD, J. C. 1961. *The Mentally Handicapped and their Families: A Social Survey* (Maudsley Monogr. No. 7). London.

365 TOKUHATA, G. K. & STEHMAN, V. A. 1961. 'Sociologic implications, and epidemiology, of mental disorders in recent Japan.' *Amer. J. publ. Hlth* 51: 697–705.

366 WHO. 1954. The Mentally Subnormal Child. *World Hlth Org. tech. Rep. Ser.* 75. Geneva.

367 WHO. 1957. *European Seminar on the Mental Health of the Subnormal Child* (Oslo, 1957). WHO Regional Office for Europe, Copenhagen.

IX. *Suicide*

368 CAPSTICK, A. 1960. 'Urban and rural suicide.' *J. ment. Sci.* **106**: 1327–36.

369 SAINSBURY, P. 1955. *Suicide in London: An Ecological Study*. London.

370 STENGEL, E. 1960. 'The complexity of motivations to suicidal attempts.' *J. ment. Sci.* **106**: 1388–93.

371 VEIL, C. 1957. 'Note sur la gravité et l'urgence en psychiatrie de dispensaire.' *Ann. médico-psychol.* **2**: 124–7.

372 YAP, P. M. 1958. *Suicide in Hong Kong*. Hong Kong.

Preventive Aspects of Mental Health Action

PROMOTION OF MENTAL HEALTH
IN THE COMMUNITY

373 CAPLAN, G. 1961. *An Approach to Community Mental Health.* London.

374 FRASER, F. 1958. 'Medical practice in a changing society.' *Lancet* 1: 154-7.

375 GOTTLIEB, J. S. & HOWELL, R. W. 1957. 'The concepts of "prevention" and "creativity development" as applied to mental health.' In *Four Basic Aspects of Preventive Psychiatry*, ed. R. H. Ojemann. State Univ. Iowa, Iowa City. Pp. 9-17.

376 JONES, K. 1960. *Mental Health and Social Policy, 1845-1959.* London. (Cf. especially Chap. 11, 'Problems and Experiments, 1948-59'; pp. 153-77.)

377 KEBRIKOV, O. V. *et al.* 1954. *Reports of the Members of the Soviet Delegation at the Fifth Congress on Mental Health Defence.* Moscow.

378 KRAPF, E. E. 1955. 'Structure and functions of the Mental Health Society.' *Ment. Hyg.* **39**: 225-31.

379 KRAPF, E. E. 1958. 'The work of the World Health Organization in relation to the mental health problems in changing cultures.' In *Growing Up in a Changing World.* WFMH, London. Pp. 106-12.

380 KRUSE, H. D. (ed.) 1957. *Integrating the Approaches to Mental Disease.* (2 Conferences held under the auspices of the Committee of Public Health, N.Y. Acad. Med.) New York.

381 LEMKAU, P. V. 1952. 'Toward mental health: Areas that promise progress.' *Ment. Hyg.* **36**: 197-209.

382 MACMILLAN, D. 1960. 'Preventive geriatrics: Opportunities of a community mental health service.' *Lancet* **2**: 1439-41.

383 SIVADON, P. & DUCHÊNE, H. 1958. 'Santé mentale, hygiène mentale et prophylaxie mentale.' In *Traité de psychiatrie: Encyclopédie médico-chirurgicale*. Paris. Tome 3, art. 37960 A30, p. 3.

384 STEVENSON, G. S. 1956. *Mental Health Planning for Social Action*. New York.

385 TUFTS, E. M. 1955. 'The field of mental health promotion.' In *Community Programs for Mental Health*, ed. R. Kotinsky & H. L. Witmer. Cambridge, Mass. Pp. 33–45.

386 WILLIAMS, C. D. 1958. 'Social medicine in developing countries.' *Lancet* I: 863–6, 919–22.

387 *Constructive Mental Hygiene in the Caribbean* (Proc. 1st Caribbean Conf. on Mental Health, March 1957). Assen.

388 MILBANK MEMORIAL FUND. 1956. *The Elements of a Community Mental Health Program*. New York. Pp. 101–5 & 122–34.
(G. R. Hargreaves: The Protection of the Personality.)

389 UNITED STATES. 1961. Joint Commission on Mental Illness and Health, *Action for Mental Health*. New York. (Cf. Summary, 'Action for Mental Health: Digest of Final Report.' *Modern Hosp.*, 1961, **96**, 109–24.)

390 WHO. 1957. The Psychiatric Hospital as a Centre for Preventive Work in Mental Health: 5th Report of the Expert Committee on Mental Health. *World Hlth Org. tech. Rep. Ser.* 134. Geneva.

391 WHO. 1961. Programme Development in the Mental Health Field: 10th Report of the Expert Committee on Mental Health. *World Hlth Org. tech. Rep. Ser.* 223. Geneva.

PUBLIC HEALTH IN ACTION

392 GRUENBERG, E. M. 1957. 'Application of control methods to mental illness.' *Amer. J. publ. Hlth.* 47: 944–52.

393 HARGREAVES, G. R. 1958. *Psychiatry and the Public Health*. London.

394 LEMKAU, P. V. 1955. *Mental Hygiene in Public Health*. (2nd ed.) New York. Pp. 11 et seq.

395 UNITED KINGDOM. 1956. *An Inquiry into Health Visiting: Report of a Working Party on the Field of Work, Training and Recruitment of Health Visitors*. Ministry of Health, Dept of Health for Scotland, and Ministry of Education, London.

LEGISLATION

396 DAVIDSON, H. A. 1959. 'The commitment procedures and their legal implications.' In *American Handbook of Psychiatry*, ed. S. Arieti. New York. Vol 2: 1902–22.

397 GOTTLIEB, J. S. & TOURNEY, G. 1958. 'Commitment procedures and the advancement of psychiatric knowledge.' *Amer. J. Psychiat.* **115**: 109–13.

398 GRAY, H. R. 1960. 'The reform of the law relating to mental health.' *New Zealand med. J.* **59**: 18–23.

399 MACLAY, W. S. 1960. 'The new Mental Health Act in England and Wales.' *Amer. J. Psychiat.* **116**: 777–81.

400 ENGLAND & WALES. 1948. *National Health Service Act, 1946: Provisions Relating to the Mental Health Services.* Ministry of Health, London.

401 SCOTLAND. 1955. *The Law Relating to Mental Illness and Mental Deficiency in Scotland: Proposals for Amendment.* Dept of Health, Edinburgh.

402 SCOTLAND. 1959. *Mental Health Legislation: 2nd Report by a Committee appointed by the Council.* Dept. of Health & Scottish Health Services Council, Edinburgh.

403 'The Mental Health Act.' 1960. *Brit. med. J.* **2**: 1297–8.

404 UNITED KINGDOM. 1957. *Royal Commission on the Law relating to Mental Illness and Mental Deficiency, 1954–1957: Report.* London.

405 WHO. 1955. *Hospitalization of Mental Patients: A Survey of Existing Legislation.* Geneva.

406 WHO. 1955. Legislation Affecting Psychiatric Treatment: 4th Report of the Expert Committee on Mental Health. *World Hlth Org. tech. Rep. Ser.* 98. Geneva.

Mental Health in Infancy

407 BOWLBY, J. 1951. *Maternal Care and Mental Health* (World Hlth Org. Monogr. Ser. 2). Geneva.

408 BOWLBY, J. 1958. 'Separation of mother and child.' *Lancet* 1: 480.

409 BOWLBY, J. 1958. 'The nature of the child's tie to his mother.' *Int. J. Psycho-Anal.* 39: 350–73.

410 FOSS, B. M. (ed.) 1961. *Determinants of Infant Behaviour: Proceedings of a Tavistock Study Group on Mother-Infant Interaction* (Ciba Foundation, Sept. 1959). London.

411 MEAD, M. 1954. 'Some theoretical considerations on the problem of mother-child separation.' *Amer. J. Orthopsychiat.* 24: 471–83.

412 MURPHY, L. B. *et al.* 1956. *Personality in Young Children.* 2 vols. New York.

413 STONE, F. H. 1958. 'Early disorders of the mother-child relationship.' *Lancet* 1: 1115–18.

414 'Problèmes d'hygiène mentale posés par la séparation des jeunes enfants de leur mère.' 1957. *Hyg. Ment.* No 1.

415 WHO. 1962. *Deprivation of Maternal Care: A Reassessment of its Effects* (World Hlth Org. publ. Hlth Papers 14). Geneva.

The Welfare of Children

416 BACKETT, E. M. & JOHNSTON, A. M. 1959. 'Social patterns of road accidents to children: Some characteristics of vulnerable families.' *Brit. med. J.* 1: 409–13.

417 BAUCHARD, P. 1953. *The Child Audience: A Report on Press, Film and Radio for Children.* UNESCO, Paris.

418 CAPLAN, G. (ed.) 1961. *Prevention of Mental Disorder in Children: Initial Explorations.* London.

419 DUHRSSEN, A. 1958. *Heimkinder und Pflegekinder in ihrer Entwicklung.* Göttingen.

420 GINZBERG, E. (ed.) 1960. *The Nation's Children.* Vols 1 & 3. New York.

421 HIMMELWEIT, H. T. *et al.* 1958. *Television and the Child.* London.

422 HOCHFELD, E. & VALK, M. A. 1953. *Experience in Inter-Country Adoptions.* Int. Social Service (Amer. Branch), New York.

423 WERTHAM, F. 1954. *Seduction of the Innocent.* New York.

424 ENGLAND & WALES. 1955. *Seventh Report on the Work of the Children's Department: November 1955.* Home Office, London.

425 ENGLAND & WALES. 1960. *Report of the Committee on Children and Young Persons.* Home Office, London.

426 UNITED KINGDOM. 1954. *Report of the Departmental Committee on the Adoption of Children.* Home Office & Scottish Home Dept, London.

427 WHO. 1953. Joint UN/WHO Meeting of Experts on the Mental Health Aspects of Adoption: Final Report. *World Hlth Org. tech. Rep. Ser.* 70. Geneva.

428 WHO. 1957. Accidents in Childhood: Facts as a Basis for Prevention – Report of an Advisory Group. *World Hlth Org. tech. Rep. Ser.* 118. Geneva.

429 WHO. 1959. 'Accidents in childhood in the Americas.' *World Hlth Org. Chron.* 13: 249–50.

430 WHO. 1960. *Seminar on the Prevention of Accidents in Childhood* (Spa, 1958). WHO Regional Office for Europe, Copenhagen.

THE FAMILY

431 ACKERMAN, N. W. *The Psychodynamics of Family Life.* New York.

432 BLACKER, C. P. 1958. 'Disruption of marriage: Some possibilities of prevention.' *Lancet* 1: 578–81.

433 EISENSTEIN, V. W. (ed.) 1956. *Neurotic Interaction in Marriage.* New York.

434 LIN, T. (ed.) 1960. *Reality and Vision: A Report of the First Asian Seminar on Mental Health and Family Life* (Baguio, 1958). Manila.

MENTAL HEALTH AND THE EDUCATIONAL SYSTEM

435 ANDERSON, H. H. *et al.* 1959. 'Image of the teacher by adolescent children in four countries: Germany, England, Mexico, United States.' *J. soc. Psychol.* **50**: 47–55.

436 BONNEY, M. E. 1960. *Mental Health in Education.* Boston.

437 BOWER, E. M. 1960. *Early Identification of Emotionally Handicapped Children in School.* Springfield, Ill.

438 KAPLAN, L. 1959. *Mental Health and Human Relations in Education.* New York.

439 KRUGMAN, M. (ed.) 1958. *Orthopsychiatry and the School.* New York.

440 MACFARLANE, J. W. 1953. 'The uses and predictive limitations of intelligence tests in infants and young children.' *Bull. World Hlth Org.* **9**: 409–15.

441 SHIPLEY, J. T. 1961. *The Mentally Disturbed Teacher.* Philadelphia.

442 WALL, W. D. 1955. *Education and Mental Health* (Problems in Education XI). UNESCO, Paris.

443 WHEELER, O., PHILLIPS, W. & SPILLANE, J. P. 1961. *Mental Health and Education.* London.

444 ENGLAND & WALES. 1952. *The Health of the School Child: Report of the Chief Medical Officer of the Ministry of Education for 1950 and 1951.* Ministry of Education, London.

445 SCOTTISH COUNCIL FOR RESEARCH IN EDUCATION. 1953. *Social Implications of the 1947 Scottish Mental Survey.*

446 SCOTTISH COUNCIL FOR RESEARCH IN EDUCATION. 1959. *Educational . . . Aspects of the 1947 Scottish Mental Survey.*

447 WHO. 1951. Expert Committee on School Health Services: Report on the 1st Session. *World Hlth Org. tech. Rep. Ser.* **30**: pp. 14–16. Geneva.

STUDENT MENTAL HEALTH

448 BLAINE, G. & MACARTHUR, C. 1961. *Emotional Problems of the Student.* New York.

449 DAVIDSON, M. A. *et al.* 1955. 'The detection of psychological vulnerability in students.' *J. ment. Sci.* **101**: 810–25.

450 DAVY, B. W. 1960. 'The sources and prevention of mental ill-health in university students.' *Proc. R. Soc. Med.* **53**: 764–9.

451 FARNSWORTH, D. L. 1957. *Mental Health in College and University*. Cambridge, Mass.

452 FARNSWORTH, D. L. 1959. 'Social and emotional development of students in college and university.' *Ment. Hyg.* **43**: 358–67, 568–76.

453 FUNKENSTEIN, D. H. (ed.) 1959. *The Student and Mental Health: An International View* (Proc. 1st Int. Conf. Student Mental Health, Princeton, 1956). Cambridge, Mass.

454 FUNKENSTEIN, D. H. & WILKIE, G. H. 1956. *Student Mental Health: An annotated Bibliography, 1936–1955.* WFMH, London; Int. Ass. Universities, Paris.

455 PRINCE, R. 1960. 'The "brain fag" syndrome in Nigerian students.' *J. ment. Sci.* **106**: 559–70.

456 ROOK, A. 1959. 'Student suicides.' *Brit. med. J.* **1**: 599–603.

457 WAGGONER, R. W. & ZEIGLER, T. W. 1961. 'Psychiatric factors in medical students in difficulty: A follow-up study.' *Amer. J. Psychiat.* **117**: 727–31.

458 WEDGE, B. M. (ed.) 1958. *Psychosocial Problems of College Men*. Div. of Student Mental Hygiene, Yale Univ.; New Haven, Conn.

459 INT. ASS. UNIVERSITIES, 1958. *Student Mental Health* (Papers Int. Ass. Universities, No. 3). Paris.

INDUSTRIAL MENTAL HEALTH

460 KOEKEBAKKER, J. 1955. 'Mental Health and Group Tensions.' *Bull. World Hlth Org.* **13**: 543–50.

461 LING, T. M. (ed.) 1954. *Mental Health and Human Relations in Industry*. London.

462 LING, T. M. 1955. 'La santé mentale dans l'industrie.' *Bull. World Hlth Org.* **13**: 551–9.

463 MINDUS, E. 1955. 'Outlines of a concept of industrial psychiatry.' *Bull. World Hlth Org.* **13**: 561–74.

464 VEIL, C. 1957. 'Aspects médico-psychologiques de l'industrialisation moderne.' *Rev. int. Travail,* **75**.
(English transl.: 'Medical and psychological aspects of modern industry.' *Int. Labour Rev.* **75**.)

465 VEIL, C. 1961. 'Hygiène mentale du travailleur.' In *Traité de psychiatrie: Encyclopédie médico-chirurgicale.* Paris. Tome 3, art. 37960 A50.

466 UNITED KINGDOM. 1958. *Final Report of the Joint Committee on Human Relations in Industry 1954–57; and Report of the Joint Committee on Individual Efficiency in Industry 1953–57.* Dept. Sci. Indust. Res. & Med. Res. Council, London.

467 WFMH. 1948. *Third International Congress on Mental Health, London 1948.* Vol. 4: *Mental Hygiene.* London. Pp. 175–209 (Mental Health in Industry and Industrial Relations).

468 WHO. 1953. Joint ILO/WHO Committee on Occupational Health: 2nd Report. *World Hlth Org. tech. Rep. Ser.* 66. Geneva.

469 WHO. 1957. Joint ILO/WHO Committee on Occupational Health: 3rd Report. *World Hlth Org. tech. Rep. Ser.* 135. Geneva.

470 WHO. 1958. *Human Relations and Mental Health in Industrial Units.* WHO Regional Office for Europe, Copenhagen.

471 WHO. 1959. Mental Health Problems of Automation: Report of a Study Group. *World Hlth Org. tech. Rep. Ser.* 183. Geneva.

PREVENTION OF CRIME AND DELINQUENCY

472 GLUECK, S. & GLUECK, E. T. 1950. *Unraveling Juvenile Delinquency.* New York.

473 GLUECK, S. & GLUECK, E. T. 1959. *Predicting Delinquency and Crime.* Cambridge, Mass.

474 GUTTMACHER, M. S. 1949. 'Medical aspects of the causes and prevention of crime and the treatment of offenders.' *Bull. World Hlth Org.* **2**: 279–88.

475 GUTTMACHER, M. S. 1950. 'Psychiatric examination of offenders.' *Bull. World Hlth Org.* **2**: 743–9.

476 LECONTE, M. 1960. 'De la nécessité de tirer quelques enseignements de l'actualité de la criminalité psychiatrique révélée par la presse.' *Ann. Méd. lég.* **40**: 246–63.

477 LOPEZ-REY, M. 1958. 'Mental health and the work of the United Nations in the field of the prevention of crime and the treatment of offenders.' In *Growing Up in a Changing World*. WFMH, London. Pp. 93–100.

478 ENGLAND & WALES. 1959. *Penal Practice in a Changing Society: Aspects of Future Development (England and Wales)*. Home Office, London.

479 ENGLAND & WALES. 1960. *Criminal Law Revision Committee: 2nd Report (Suicide)*. Home Office, London.

480 UN DEPT. OF SOCIAL AFFAIRS. 1953. *Int. Rev. crim. Policy*. Special issue on Medical, Psychological, and Social Examination of Offenders.

481 UN DEPT. OF SOCIAL AFFAIRS. 1959. European Consultative Group on the Prevention of Crime and Treatment of Offenders (4th Session, Geneva, 1958). *Int. Rev. crim. Policy* **14**: 59–69.

482 UNESCO. 1957. *The University Teaching of Social Sciences: Criminology*. Paris.

Social and Cross-cultural Aspects
of Mental Health Action

HEALTH AND HUMAN WELFARE

483 BURGESS, A. & DEAN, R. F. A. (eds.) 1962. *Malnutrition and Food Habits* (Report of an International and Interprofessional Conference, Cuernavaca, Mexico, 1960). London.

484 FELIX, R. H. *et al.* 1961. *Mental Health and Social Welfare.* New York.

485 MEERLOO, J. A. M. 1952. 'Contribution of the psychiatrist to the management of crisis situations.' *Amer. J. Psychiat.* **109**: 352–5.

486 OPLER, M. K. (ed.) 1959. *Culture and Mental Health: Cross-cultural Studies.* New York.

487 PETRULLO, L. & BASS, B. M. (eds.) 1961. *Leadership and Interpersonal Behavior.* New York.

488 RUBIN, V. (ed.) 1960. *Culture, Society and Health.* New York.

489 WELFORD, A. T. *et al.* (eds.) 1962. *Society: Problems and Methods of Study.* London.

490 JOSIAH MACY, JR FOUNDATION. 1950. *Health and Human Relations in Germany.* New York.

491 JOSIAH MACY, JR FOUNDATION. 1951. *Health and Human Relations in Germany.* New York.

492 *Research into Factors Influencing Human Relations: Report of the International Conference (Nijmegen).* Hilversum, 1956.

493 WFMH. 1959. *Africa: Social Change and Mental Health – Report of a Panel Discussion.* . . . (New York, 23 March 1959). London.

CULTURAL STUDIES

494 BIESHEUVEL, S. 1960. 'Select bibliography on the aptitude of the African south of the Sahara, 1917–1958.' In *Mental*

335

Disorders and Mental Health in Africa South of the Sahara,
CCTA/CSA Publ. No. 35. London. Pp. 263–9.

495 CAROTHERS, J. C. 1953. *The African Mind in Health and Disease: A Study in Ethnopsychiatry* (World Hlth Org. Monogr. Ser. 17). Geneva.

496 DUBOIS, J. A. 1906. *Hindu Manners, Customs and Ceremonies* (transl. from the French MS (1806) and ed. H. K. Beauchamp). (3rd ed.) Oxford. Pp. 160, 522–41.

497 GEBER, M. & DEAN, R. F. A. 1958. 'Psychomotor development in African children: The effects of social class and the need for improved tests.' *Bull. World Hlth Org.* 18: 471–6.

498 HOFFET, F. 1951. *Psychanalyse de l'Alsace*. Paris.

499 HSU, F. L. K. (ed.) 1961. *Psychological Anthropology: Approaches to Culture and Personality*. Homewood, Illinois.

500 HUGHES, C. C. 1960. *An Eskimo Village in the Modern World*. Ithaca, N.Y.

501 KAPLAN, B. (ed.) 1961. *Studying Personality Cross-culturally*. New York.

502 LA BARRE, W. 1962. *They shall take up Serpents: Psychology of the Southern Snake-handling Cult*. Minneapolis. P. 160.

503 LIPSET, S. M. & LOWENTHAL, L. (eds.) 1961. *Culture and Social Character: The Work of David Riesman Reviewed*. New York.

504 MEAD, M. (ed.) 1953. *Cultural Patterns and Technical Change*. UNESCO, Paris.

505 MEAD, M. 1956. *New Lives for Old: Cultural Transformation – Manus, 1928–1953*. London.

506 MEAD, M. 1959. *An Anthropologist at Work: Writings of Ruth Benedict*. Boston.

507 MEAD, M. & WOLFENSTEIN, M. (eds.) 1955 & 1962. *Childhood in Contemporary Cultures*. Chicago.

508 MEADE, J. E. *et al.* 1961. *The Economic and Social Structure of Mauritius*. London.

509 OPLER, M. K. 1956. 'Ethnic differences in behaviour and psychopathology: Italian and Irish.' *Int. J. soc. Psychiat.* 2: 11–22.

510 SODDY, K. (ed.) 1955–56. *Mental Health and Infant Develop-ment* (Proc. WFMH Int. Seminar, Chichester, 1952). Vol. 1: *Papers and Discussions*; Vol. 2: *Case Histories*. 2 vols. London & New York.

511 WAGLEY, C. (ed.) 1952. *Race and Class in Rural Brazil*. UNESCO, Paris.

512 CCTA/CSA. 1960. *CSA Meeting of Specialists on the Basic Psychology of African and Madagascan Populations* (Tananarive, 1959). Publ. No. 51. London.

SOME SOCIAL QUESTIONS

I. *Ageing*

513 TIBBITTS, C. (ed.) 1960. *Handbook of Social Gerontology: Social Aspects of Aging*. Chicago.

514 TIBBITTS, C. & DONAHUE, W. (eds.) 1960. *Aging in Today's Society*. New Jersey.

515 TOWNSEND, P. 1959. 'Social surveys of old age in Great Britain 1945–58.' *Bull. World Hlth Org.* **21**: 583–91.

II. *Industrialization and Urbanization*

516 CLAY, H. M. 1960. *The Older Worker and his Job* (Problems of Progress in Industry, No. 7). London.

517 CROOME, H. 1960. *Human Problems of Innovation* (Problems of Progress in Industry, No. 5). London.

518 FRIEDMAN, G. 1955. *Industrial Society: The Emergence of the Human Problems of Automation*. Glencoe, Ill.

519 RODGER, A. 1959. 'Ten years of ergonomics.' *Nature, Lond.*, **184**: 20–2.

520 SCOTT, J. F. & LYNTON, R. P. 1952. *The Community Factor in Modern Technology*. UNESCO, Paris.

521 THOMSON, D. C. (ed.) 1957. *Management, Labour and Community*, London.

522 VEIL, C. 1957. 'Phénoménologie du travail.' *Evolut. psychiat.* **4**: 693–721.

523 WELFORD, A. T. 1960. *Ergonomics of Automation* (Problems of Progress in Industry, No. 8). London.

524 CARNEGIE STUDY GROUP. 1958. 'Proceedings of the Carnegie Study Group on the basic principles of automation (Geneva, 1957).' *Int. soc. Sci. Bull.* 10: 1.

525 ILO. 1961. 'Ergonomics: The scientific approach to making work human.' *Int. Labour Rev.* 83: 1–35.

526 UNESCO. 1956. *The Social Implications of Industrialization and Urbanization in Africa South of the Sahara.* Paris.

527 UNESCO. 1956. *The Social Implications of Industrialization and Urbanization: Five Studies of Urban Populations of Recent Rural Origin in Cities of Southern Asia.* Calcutta.

528 UNITED KINGDOM. 1956. *Automation: A Report on the Technical Trends and their Impact on Management and Labour.* Dept. Sci. Industr. Res., London.

529 UNITED KINGDOM. 1957. *Men, Steel and Technical Change* (Problems of Progress in Industry, No. 1). London.

530 UNITED KINGDOM. 1960. *Woman, Wife and Worker* (Problems of Progress in Industry, No. 10). London.

531 WFMH. 1957. *Mental Health Aspects of Urbanisation* (Report of discussions conducted in the Economic & Social Council Chamber, United Nations, New York, 1957, by WFMH). London.

532 WHO. 1958. Mental Health Aspects of the Peaceful Uses of Atomic Energy: Report of a Study Group. *World Hlth Org. tech. Rep. Ser.* 151. Geneva.

533 WHO. 1960. 'The psycho-social environment in industry.' *World Hlth Org. Chron.* 14: 276–9.

III. *International Action*

534 BERGER, G. *et al.* 1959. 'Rapports de l'Occident avec le reste du monde.' *Perspectives*, Paris, No. 3 (avril). (Cf. English review: *World ment. Hlth* 1959, 11: 190–5.)

535 KISKER, G. W. (ed.) 1951. *World Tensions: The Psychopathology of International Relations.* New York.

536 OPLER, M. E. 1954. *Social Aspects of Technical Assistance in Operation.* UNESCO, Paris.

537 UNESCO. 1953. *Interrelations of Cultures: Their Contribution to International Understanding.* Paris.

538 UNESCO. 1957. *The Nature of Conflict: Studies on the Sociological Aspects of International Tensions.* Paris.

539 WFMH. 1955. *Social Implications of Technical Assistance* (Report of a meeting held at the UN, New York, 1955). London.

IV. *Migration and Social Displacement*

540 BORRIE, W. D. *et al.* 1959. *The Cultural Integration of Immigrants.* UNESCO, Paris.

541 CURLE, A. & TRIST, E. 1947. 'Transitional communities and social reconnection.' *Human Relations* **1**: 42–68, 240–288.

542 MURPHY, H. B. M. *et al.* 1955. *Flight and Resettlement.* UNESCO, Paris.

543 ILO. 1959. *International Migration, 1945–1957* (Studies and Reports, No. 54). Geneva.

544 ILO. 1961. 'Some aspects of the international migration of families.' *Int. Labour Rev.* **83**: 65–86.

545 WFMH. 1960. *Uprooting and Resettlement* (11th Ann. Meeting WFMH, Vienna, 1958). London.

V. *Population*

546 LORIMER, F. *et al.* 1954. *Culture and Human Fertility.* UNESCO, Paris.

547 PINCUS, G. 1961. 'Suppression of ovulation with reference to oral contraceptives.' In *Modern Trends in Endocrinology*, 2nd ser., ed. H. Gardiner-Hill. London. Pp. 231–45.

548 TITMUSS, R. M. & ABEL SMITH, B. 1961. *Social Policies and Population Growth in Mauritius.* London.

549 'Mauritius and Malthus.' 1961. *Lancet* **1**: 542–3.

550 UNITED KINGDOM. 1960. *Report of the Departmental Committee on Human Artificial Insemination.* Home Office & Scottish Home Dept, London.

SOME SOCIAL DIFFICULTIES

I. *Delinquency*

551 ERIKSON, E. H. 1956. *New Perspectives for Research on Juvenile Delinquency.* Washington, D.C.

552 WILKINS, L. T. 1960. *Delinquent Generations.* London.

553 UN DEPT. OF ECON. SOCIAL AFFAIRS (DIV. OF SOCIAL WELFARE). 1952–58. *Comparative Survey on Juvenile Delinquency.* Pt I: North America (revised ed.); Pt II: Europe (in French*); Pt III: Latin America (revised ed.) (in Spanish**); Pt IV: Asia and the Far East; Pt V: Middle East. New York.
(*English summary in *Int. Rev. crim. Policy*, 1954, No. 5: 19–38.)
(**Cf. also J. A. Smythe, 'Juvenile delinquency in Latin American countries.' *Int. Rev. crim. Policy*, 1954, No. 5: 9–18.)

II. *Pathological Attitudes and Mental Disorder*

554 CARSTAIRS, G. M. 1958. 'Some problems of psychiatry in patients from alien cultures.' *Lancet* 1: 1217–20.

555 EISLER, R. 1951. *Man into Wolf: An Anthropological Interpretation of Sadism, Masochism and Lycanthropy.* London.

556 FIELD, M. J. 1955. 'Witchcraft as a primitive interpretation of mental disorder.' *J. ment. Sci.* 101: 826–33.
(Cf. also *J. ment. Sci.* 108: 1043.)

557 GILLIS, L. 1962. *Human Behaviour in Illness: Psychology and Interpersonal Relationships.* With a contribution by S. Biesheuvel. London.

558 JUNG, C. G. 1959. *Flying Saucers: A Modern Myth of Things seen in the Skies* (transl. R. F. C. Hull). London.

559 MEERLOO, J. A. M. 1957. *Mental Seduction and Menticide: The Psychology of Thought Control and Brainwashing.* London.

560 MEERLOO, J. A. M. 1958. ' "Infection mentale": Communication archaïque et régression insensible – Contribution à l'étude psychosomatique des épidémies mentales.' *Méd. et Hyg., Genève,* **16**: 469 et seq.

561 MEERLOO, J. A. M. 1958. 'The delusion of the flying saucer.' *Amer. Practitioner* **9**: 1631–6.

562 MEERLOO, J. A. M. 1959. 'Rock 'n roll: A modern aspect of St Vitus dance – implications for the theory of mental contagion.' *Amer. Practitioner* **10**: 1029–32.

563 SARGANT, W. 1957. *Battle for the Mind: A Physiology of Conversion and Brain-Washing.* London.

564 STENGEL, E. & COOK, N. G. 1958. *Attempted Suicide: Its Social Significance and Effects* (Maudsley Monogr. No. 4). London.

565 WITTKOWER, E. D. & FRIED, J. 1959. 'A cross-cultural approach to mental health problems.' *Amer. J. Psychiat.* **116**: 423–8.

566 CHURCH [OF ENGLAND] ASSEMBLY BOARD FOR SOCIAL RESPONSIBILITY. 1959. *Ought Suicide to be a Crime? – A Discussion of Suicide, Attempted Suicide and the Law.* London.

567 MILBANK MEMORIAL FUND. 1953. *Interrelations between the Social Environment and Psychiatric Disorders.* New York.

III. *Prejudice and Discrimination*

568 ADORNO, T. W. *et al.* 1950. *The Authoritarian Personality.* New York.

569 ALLPORT, G. W. 1954. *The Nature of Prejudice.* Cambridge, Mass.

570 BIESHEUVEL, S. 1959. *Race, Culture and Personality.* Johannesburg.

571 MYERS, J. K. & ROBERTS, B. 1959. *Family and Class Dynamics.* London.

572 GROUP FOR THE ADVANCEMENT OF PSYCHIATRY (GAP). 1957. *Psychological Aspects of School Desegregation* (Report No. 37). New York.

573 UNESCO. 1956. *The Race Question in Modern Science.* Paris.

IV. *Problems of Sex Behaviour*

574 ALLEN, C. 1958. *Homosexuality: Its Nature, Causation and Treatment.* London. (Cf. especially Pt. III: 'Social Significance'; pp. 54–63.)

575 BAILEY, D. S. (ed.) 1956. *Sexual Offenders and Social Punishment.* Church of England Moral Welfare Council, London.

576 FORD, C. S. & BEACH, F. A. 1951. *Patterns of Sexual Behavior.* New York.

577 WESTWOOD, G. 1960. *A Minority: A Report of the Life of the Male Homosexual in Great Britain.* London.

578 BRITISH MEDICAL ASS. 1955. *Homosexuality and Prostitution.* London.

579 UNITED KINGDOM. 1957. *Report of the Committee on Homosexual Offences and Prostitution.* Home Office, Scottish Home Dept, London.

Professional Training

Psychiatry and the Medical Undergraduate

580 BALINT, M. 1961. 'The pyramid and the psychotherapeutic relationship.' (Re: Training of medical students.) *Lancet* 2: 1051–4.

581 BARTON HALL, S., HEARNSHAW, L. S. & HETHERINGTON, R. R. 1961. 'The teaching of psychology in the medical curriculum.' *J. ment. Sci.* 107: 1003–10.

582 CURRAN, D. 1955. 'The place of psychology and psychiatry in medical education.' *Brit. med. J.* 2: 515–18.

583 HARGREAVES, G. R., BROWN, D. G. & WHYTE, M. B. H. 1962. 'Home visits by medical students: An aspect of psychiatric education.' *Lancet* 2: 141–2.

584 HENDERSON, D. 1955. 'Why psychiatry?' *Brit. med. J.* 2: 519–23.

585 HILL, D. 1960. 'Acceptance of psychiatry by the medical student.' *Brit. med. J.* 1: 917–18.

586 LEVINE, M. & LEDERER, H. D. 1959. 'Teaching of psychiatry in medical schools.' In *American Handbook of Psychiatry*, ed. S. Arieti. New York. Vol. 2: 1923–34.

587 MACCALMAN, D. R. 1953. 'Observations on the teaching of the principles of mental health to medical students' (and Memorandum on undergraduate teaching of psychiatry – from the Roy. Med.-Psychol. Ass.). *Brit. J. med. Psychol.* 26: 140–51.

588 PARKER, S. 1960. 'The attitudes of medical students toward their patients: An exploratory study.' *J. med. Educ.* 35: 849–56.

589 RICKLES, N. K. 1960. 'General medicine before specialization.' *Amer. J. Psychiat.* 116: 663.

590 STEVENSON, I. 1961. *Medical History-taking.* New York.

591 TANNER, J. M. 1958. 'The place of human biology in medical education.' *Lancet* 1: 1185–8.

592 TREDGOLD, R. F. 1962. 'The integration of psychiatric teaching into the curriculum.' *Lancet* 1. 1344–7.

593 AMERICAN PSYCHIATRIC ASS. 1952. *Psychiatry and Medical Education.* Washington, D.C.

594 'Psychological medicine and undergraduate education.' 1958. *Brit. med. J.* 2: 602.

595 WHO. 1961. The Undergraduate Teaching of Psychiatry and Mental Health Promotion: 9th Report of the Expert Committee on Mental Health. *World Hlth Org. tech. Rep. Ser.* 208. Geneva.

596 WHO. 1961. *Teaching of Psychiatry and Mental Health* (World Hlth Org. publ. Hlth Papers 9). Geneva.

PSYCHIATRY AND THE MEDICAL POSTGRADUATE

597 BLEULER, M. *et al.* 1961. *Teaching of Psychiatry and Mental Health* (World Hlth Org. publ. Hlth Papers 9). Geneva.

598 DAVIES, T. T., DAVIES, E. T. L. & O'NEILL, D. 1958. 'Case-work in the teaching of psychiatry.' *Lancet* 2: 34–7.

599 GILDEA, E. F. 1959. 'Teaching of psychiatry to residents.' In *American Handbook of Psychiatry*, ed. S. Arieti. New York. Vol. 2: 1935–47.

600 HOLT, R. R. & LUBORSKY, L. 1958. *Personality Patterns of Psychiatrists: A Study of Methods of Selecting Residents.* New York.

601 LEVY, D. M. 1959. *The Demonstration Clinic for the Psychological Study and Treatment of Mother and Child in Medical Practice.* Springfield, Ill.

602 MEARES, A. 1960. 'Communication with the patient.' *Lancet* 1: 663–7.

603 AMERICAN PSYCHIATRIC ASS. 1953. *The Psychiatrist: His Training and Development.* Washington, D.C.

604 ROYAL MEDICO-PSYCHOL. ASS. 1951. *Memorandum on the Training of the Consultant Child Psychiatrist.* London.

605 ROYAL MEDICO-PSYCHOL. ASS. 1960. *The Recruitment and Training of the Child Psychiatrist.* London.

(Cf. Recruitment and training of child psychiatrists. *Brit. med. J.*, 1960. **2**: 205–6.)

PSYCHIATRY AND THE GENERAL PRACTITIONER

606 BALINT, M. 1954. 'Training general practitioners in psychotherapy.' *Brit. med. J.* **1**: 115–20.

607 CARSTAIRS, G. M., WALTON, H. J. & FAWCETT, P. G. 1962. 'General practitioners and psychological medicine: Their views on a postgraduate course.' *Lancet* **2**: 397.

608 GOSHEN, C. E. 1959. 'A project for the creation of better understanding of psychiatry by the general practitioner.' *Southern med. J.* **52**: 30–4.

OTHER PROFESSIONAL TRAINING IN THE MENTAL HEALTH FIELD

609 AFFLECK, J. W. *et al.* 1960. 'In-service mental-health teaching for health visitors.' *Lancet* **2**: 641–3.

610 CAPLAN, G. 1959. 'An approach to the education of community mental health specialists.' *Ment. Hyg.* **43**: 268–80.

611 FERARD, M. L. & HUNNYBUN, N. K. 1962. *The Caseworker's Use of Relationships*. London.

612 JAMES, E. 1958. 'The education of the scientist.' *Brit. med. J.* **2**: 575–6.

613 WRIGHT, M. S. 1962. *An Interim Report on the Characteristics of Successful and Unsuccessful Student Nurses in Scotland*. Edinburgh.
(*As summarized:* Intelligence and student nurses. *Brit. med. J.*, 1962, **2**: 37–8.)

614 AMERICAN ASS. PSYCHIAT. SOCIAL WORKERS. 1950. *Education for Psychiatric Social Work*. New York.

615 (BRITISH) ASS. PSYCHIAT. SOCIAL WORKERS. 1957. *Essentials of Case Work*. London.

616 ENGLAND & WALES. 1962. *The Training of Staff of Training Centres for the Mentally Subnormal*. Ministry of Health

(Central Health Services Council Standing Mental Health Advisory Committee), London.

617 LEVERHULME STUDY GROUP. 1961. *The Complete Scientist: An Inquiry into the Problem of achieving Breadth in the Education at School and University of Scientists, Engineers and other Technologists* (Report of the Leverhulme Study Group to the Brit. Ass. Advance. Sci.). London.

618 'Papers on the Teaching of Personality Development.' 1958. *Sociol. Rev. Monogr.* No. 1.

619 WFMH. 1956. *Mental Health in Teacher Education.* London.

620 WHO. 1956. Expert Committee on Psychiatric Nursing: 1st Report. *World Hlth Org. tech. Rep. Ser.* 105. Geneva.

AUDIO-VISUAL AIDS

621 PILKINGTON, T. L. 1960. 'The use of film in psychiatry.' *World ment. Hlth* 12: 143–5.

622 RUHE, D. S. *et al.* 1960. 'Television in the teaching of psychiatry: Report of four years' preliminary development.' *J. med. Educ.* 35: 916–26.

623 STAFFORD-CLARK, D. *et al.* 1961. 'Television in medical education.' *Brit. med. J.* 1: 500.

CATALOGUES OF FILMS FOR PSYCHIATRIC, PROFESSIONAL, AND PUBLIC EDUCATION:

624 (*a*) Deutsches Zentralinstitut für Lehrmittel. 1960. *Verzeichnis der wissenschaftlichen Filme.* Berlin (East Germany).

625 (*b*) Institut für den wissenschaftlichen Film. 1960. *Gesamtverzeichnis der wissenschaftlichen Filme.* Göttingen (German Federal Republic).

626 (*c*) La Presse Médicale. 1956–57. *Films médicaux et chirurgicaux français*, ed. P. Détrie. Paris, 1956; Supplément, 1957.

627 (*d*) Scientific Film Ass. 1960. *Films of Psychology and Psychiatry.* London.

628   (*e*) U.S. Information Agency. 1956. *United States Educational, Scientific, and Cultural Motion Pictures and Filmstrips: Science Section*. Washington, D.C.

629   (*f*) WFMH. 1960. *International Catalogue of Mental Health Films*, ed. T. L. Pilkington. (2nd ed.) London.

Public Education in Mental Health

PROGRAMMES AND THEIR EVALUATION

630 MEAD, M. 1959. 'Cultural factors in community-education programs.' In *Community Education Principles and Practices from World-wide Experience* (58th Yearbook of the Nat. Soc. for the Study of Education), ed. N. B. Henry. Chicago.

631 POWELL, E. 1961. Everybody's business: Emerging patterns for mental health services and the public (NAMH London Ann. Conf.). As reported in *Brit. med. J.* 1: 820. (Cf. *Lancet* 1: 608–9.)

632 RIDENOUR, N. 1953. 'Criteria of effectiveness in mental health education.' *Amer. J. Orthopsychiat.* 23: 271–9.

633 PENNSYLVANIA MENTAL HEALTH, INC. 1960. *Mental Health Education: A Critique*. Philadelphia.

634 WHO. 1958. Expert Committee on Training of Health Personnel in Health Education of the Public. *World Hlth Org. tech. Rep. Ser.* 156. Geneva.

635 WHO. 1959. Conference on Mental Hygiene Practice (Helsinki, 1959). Report of Committee C: The Education of the Public in Mental Health Principles. WHO Regional Office for Europe, Copenhagen. (Duplicated document.)

PROGRAMMES FOR PARENTS

636 ISAMBERT, A. 1960. *L'Education des parents*. Paris.

637 ISAMBERT, A. 1960. 'Parent education in France.' *World ment. Hlth* 12: 130–3.

638 LEWIS, R. S., STRAUSS, A. A. & LEHTINEN, L. E. 1960. *The Brain-Injured Child: A Book for Parents and Laymen*. (2nd ed.) London.

639 MACKAY, J. L. 1960. 'Parent education in the United States of America.' *World ment. Hlth* 12: 76–85.

640 STERN, H. H. 1960. *Parent Education: An International Survey.* Univ. of Hull, & UNESCO Inst. for Education. Hull.

641 LOUISIANA ASS. MENTAL HEALTH. 1957. *The New Revised and Extended 'Pierre the Pelican' Series.* 28 issues. New Orleans.

POPULAR CONCEPTS OF MENTAL HEALTH

642 CARSTAIRS, G. M. & WING, J. K. 1958. 'Attitudes of the general public to mental illness.' *Brit. med. J.* **2**: 594–7.

643 LEMKAU, P. V. & CROCETTI, G. M. 1962. 'An urban population's opinion and knowledge about mental illness.' *Amer. J. Psychiat.* **118**: 692–700.

644 NUNNALLY, J. C., JR. 1961. *Popular Conceptions of Mental Health: Their Development and Change.* New York.

645 PAUL, B. D. (ed.) 1955. *Health, Culture and Community: Case Studies of Public Reactions to Health Programs.* New York.

USE OF THE MASS MEDIA

646 ESSEX-LOPRESTI, M. 1961. 'National television programmes.' *Med. biol. Illustr.* **11**: 68.

647 JACOBY, A. 1960. 'On using mental health films.' In *International Catalogue of Mental Health Films.* (2nd ed.) WFMH, London. Pp. 6–7.

648 AMERICAN PSYCHIATRIC ASS. 1956. *Psychiatry, the Press and the Public: Problems in Communication.* Washington, D.C.

649 WHO. 1959. *World Health* **12**, No. 3 (May–June 1959). Special issue: Mental Health.

650 WHO. 1961. *World Health* **14**, No. 4 (July–Aug. 1961). To counter mental illness: Science. A special issue to mark the conclusion of the Mental Health Year (1960–61).

Additional References

651 KAY, D. & ROTH, M. 1961. 'Physical disability and emotional factors in the mental disorders.' Paper read at the IIIrd World Congress of Psychiatry, Montreal, June 1961.

652 SELLIN, T. 1938. 'Culture conflict and crime.' *Soc. Sci. Res. Bull.* **41**; *Am. J. Sociol.* **44**: 97–103.

653 BOWLBY, J. 1960. 'Grief and mourning in infancy and early childhood.' *Psycho-Anal. Study Child* **15**: 9–52.

654 BOWLBY, J. 1961. 'Processes of mourning.' *Int. J. Psycho-Anal.* **42**: 317–40.

655 BOWLBY, J. 1961. 'Childhood mourning and its implications for psychiatry.' *Am. J. Psychiat.* **118**: 481.

656 BUCKLE, D. F. 1962. 'Quelques aspects de l'évolution de la pratique psychiatrique en Europe.' *L'information psychiatrique* **5**: No. 5.

    (in English: 'Some developments of psychiatric practice in Europe.' 1962. *Aust. Psychiat. Bull.* **3**: Nos. 3 & 4.

    in Czech: 'K Vyvoji psychiatrické praxe v Evrope.' 1963. *Cs. Psychiat.* **59**.

    in Greek: 'Exelixis tinés ton efarmogon tis psykiatrikis is tin Evropin.' *Arch. med. Sci.*, Athens, 1962, No. 2.)

657 ZIER, A. & DOSHAY, L. J. 1957. 'Procyclidine hydrochloride ("Kemadrin") treatment of parkinsonism.' *Neurology* **7**: 485–9.

658 SCHWAB, R. S. 1959. 'Problems in the treatment of Parkinson's disease in elderly patients.' *Geriatrics* **14**: 545–58.

659 LINDSAY, T. F. 1961. 'When scientists stop being human.' *Daily Telegraph*, London, 19 January.

660 PENROSE, L. S. 1959. 'The somatic chromosomes in mongolism.' *Lancet* **1**: 710.

661 KORZYBSKI. 1927. *Science and Sanity*.

662 KORZYBSKI. 1931. *Un système non-aristotélien et sa nécessité pour la rigeur en mathématique et en physique.* Communication to the Congress of the American Mathematical Society, New Orleans.

663 MOUNIER, E. 1949. *Le personnalisme.* Paris. Pp. 8–10. (English transl. *Personalism.* London, 1952.)

664 JAQUES, E. 1951. *The Changing Culture of a Factory.* London.

665 PASAMANICK, B. & LILIENFELD, A. M. 1955. 'The association of maternal and foetal factors with the development of mental deficiency.' *J.A.M.A.* **159**: 155–60.

666 STAR, SHIRLEY. 1952. *Attitudes to Mental Illness.* Chicago: National Opinion Research Center Study. (Mimeographed.)

667 RIESMAN, D. 1950. *The Lonely Crowd.* New Haven.

668 MAIN, T. F. 1958. 'Some thoughts on group behaviour.' Paper read at the Davidson Clinic Summer School, Edinburgh, 1958. (Unpublished.)

669 SIGERIST, H. E. 1945. *Civilization and Disease.* New York. Pp. 66–71.

670 CURRAN, D. 1952. 'Psychiatry Ltd.' *J. ment. Sci.* **98**: 373–81.

671 TREDGOLD, R. F. & SODDY, K. 1963. *Tredgold's Textbook of Mental Deficiency.* (10th edition.) London. Pp. 98 and 151–229.

672 MIDDENDORF, W. 1960. *New Forms of Juvenile Delinquency: their Origin, Prevention and Treatment* (2nd UN Congress Prev. Crime & Treat. Offenders). UN Dept. Econ. Social Affairs, New York.

673 LEBOVICI, S. 1959. 'La prévention en santé mentale chez l'enfant.' Réflexions à propos du Seminar de Copenhague sous les auspices de l'Organisation mondiale de la Santé, 1958. *Psychiatrie de l'Enfant* **2**: 197–226.

674 ENGEL, G. L. 1961. 'Is grief a disease?' *Psychosomat. Med.* **23**: 18–22.

675 SPITZ, R. 1945. *The Psychoanalytic Study of the Child* **1**: 53. ibid. 1946, **2**: 113.

Supplementary Titles

ABRAMS, A., TOMAN, J. E. P. & GARNER, H. H. 1963. *Unfinished Tasks in the Behavioral Sciences*. London.

ALLINSMITH, W. & GOETHALS, G. W. 1962. *The Role of Schools in Mental Health*. New York.

APLEY, J. & MACKEITH, R. 1962. *The Child and his Symptoms*. Oxford.

ATKIN, I. 1962. *Aspects of Psychotherapy*. Edinburgh.

BARTON, WALTER. 1962. *Administration in Psychiatry*. Springfield, Illinois.

BOCKHOVEN, J. S. 1963. *Moral Treatment in American Psychiatry*. New York.

BOSCH, GERHARD. 1962. *Der Frühkindliche Autismus*. Berlin, Göttingen, Heidelberg.

CLARK, D. H. 1964. *Administrative Therapy*. London.

COHEN, JOHN. (ed.) 1964. *Readings in Psychology*. London.

CURRAN, D. & PARTRIDGE, M. 1963. *Psychological Medicine*. Edinburgh.

DAVIES, E. B. (ed.) 1964. *Depression* (Proceedings of a symposium by the Cambridge Postgraduate Medical School). London.

DUHL, L. J. (ed.) 1963. *The Urban Condition. People and Policy in the Metropolis*. New York.

EPSTEIN, C. 1962. *Intergroup Relations for Police Officers*. London.

FISH, F. J. 1963. *Clinical Psychiatry for the Layman*. Bristol.

FISH, F. J. 1964. *An Outline of Psychiatry for Students and Practitioners*. Bristol.

FREEMAN, H. E. & SIMMONS, O. G. 1963. *The Mental Patient comes Home*. New York.

GETZELS, J. W. & JACKSON, P. W. 1962. *Creativity and Intelligence: Explorations with Gifted Students*. New York.

GIBSON, J. 1962. *Psychiatry for Nurses*. Oxford.

352

GIBSON, J. 1963. *A Guide to Psychiatry*. Oxford.

GILBERT, J. B. 1962. *Disease and Destiny*. London.

GOLDFARB, W. 1961. *Childhood Schizophrenia*. Cambridge, Mass.

HALLAS, C. H. 1962. *Nursing the Mentally Subnormal*. Bristol.

HEATON-WARD, W. A. 1963. *Mental Subnormality*. (2nd ed.) Bristol.

HOLMES, D. J. 1963. *The Adolescent in Psychotherapy*. London.

HOWELLS, J. G. 1963. *Family Psychiatry*. Edinburgh.

ILLINGWORTH, R. S. 1963. *The Normal School Child: His Problems, Physical and Emotional*. London.

JOHN, A. L. 1961. *A Study of the Psychiatric Nurse*. Edinburgh.

JOHNSTON, N., SAVITZ, L. & WOLFGANG, M. E. (eds.) 1962. *The Sociology of Punishment and Correction: A Book of Readings*. New York.

JONES, M. 1962. *Social Psychiatry: in the Community, in Hospitals and in Prisons*. Springfield, Illinois.

KAPLAN, M. 1960. *Leisure in America: a social inquiry*. New York.

KELLNER, R. 1963. *Family Ill Health*. London.

KRAKOWSKI, A. J. & SANTORA, D. A. 1962. *Child Psychiatry and the General Practitioner*. Illinois.

KRAMER, B. M. 1962. *Day Hospital*. New York.

LEIGHTON, A. H. *et al*. 1963. *Psychiatric Disorder among the Yoruba*. New York.

LIN, TSUNG-YI & STANDLEY, C. C. 1962. *The Scope of Epidemiology in Psychiatry* (World Hlth Org. publ. Hlth Papers 16). Geneva.

MACKENZIE, M. 1963. *Psychological Depression: A Common Disorder of Personality*. London.

MADDISON, D. C. 1963. *Psychiatric Nursing*. Edinburgh.

MARKS, P. A. & SEEMAN, W. 1963. *The Actuarial Description of Abnormal Personality*. London.

MCGHIE, A. 1963. *Psychology as applied to Nursing*. Edinburgh.

MOWBRAY, R. M. & RODGER, T. F. 1963. *Psychology in relation to Medicine*. Edinburgh.

OLMSTEAD, C. 1962. *Heads I win, Tails you lose*. New York.

353

PRONKO, N. H. 1963. *Textbook of Abnormal Psychology*. London.

PUGH, T. F. 1962. *Epidemiologic Findings in United States Mental Hospital Data*. London.

RICHTER, D., TANNER, J. M., TAYLOR, LORD & ZANGWILL, O. L. (eds.) 1962. *Aspects of Psychiatric Research*. London.

RIDENOUR, NINA. 1961. *Mental Health in the United States*. Harvard.

RODGER, T. F., INGRAM, I. M. & MOWBRAY, R. M. 1962. *Lecture Notes on Psychological Medicine*. Edinburgh.

SARGANT, W. & SLATER, E. 1963. *An Introduction to Physical Methods of Treatment in Psychiatry*. Edinburgh.

SARASON, S., DAVIDSON, K. & BLATT, B. 1962. *The Preparation of Teachers*. New York.

SCHIMEL, J. L. 1961. *How to be an Adolescent – and Survive*. New York.

SIM, M. 1963. *Guide to Psychiatry*. Edinburgh.

STAFFORD-CLARK, D. 1964. *Psychiatry for Students*. London.

STEINFELD, J. I. 1963. *A New Approach to Schizophrenia*. London.

TAYLOR, LORD & CHAVE, S. 1964. *Mental Health and Environment*. London.

THOMPSON, G. G. 1962. *Child Psychology*. London.

VALENTINE, M. *An Introduction to Psychiatry*. Edinburgh.

WAHL, C. W. 1963. *Psychosomatic Medicine*. London.

WEINBERG, A. A. 1961. *Migration and Belonging. A Study of Mental Health and Personal Adjustment in Israel*. The Hague.

WELFORD, A. T., ARGYLE, M., GLASS, D. V. & MORRIS, J. N. (eds.) 1962. *Society: Problems and Methods of Study*. New York.

WENAR, C., HANDLON, M. W. & GARNER, A. M. 1962. *Psychosomatic and Emotional Disturbances: A Study of Mother-Child-Relationships* (A Psychosomatic Medicine Monograph). New York.

WOLFGANG, M. E., SAVITZ, L. & JOHNSTON, N. (eds.) 1962. *The Sociology of Crime and Delinquency: a Book of Readings*. New York.

ZILBOORG, G. 1962. *Psychoanalysis and Religion.* New York.

VAN ZONNEVELD, R. J. 1961. *The Health of the Aged.* Edinburgh.

ASSOCIATION OF THE BAR OF THE CITY OF NEW YORK WITH CORNELL UNIVERSITY LAW SCHOOL. 1962. *Mental Illness and Due Process.* New York.

GROUP FOR THE ADVANCEMENT OF PSYCHIATRY (GAP), COMMITTEE ON HOSPITALS. 1963. *Public Relations: A Responsibility of the Mental Hospital Administration.* New York.

Proceedings of the Third World Congress of Psychiatry, Montreal. 1961. Vols I & II. Toronto and Montreal.

ROYAL MEDICO-PSYCHOL. ASS. 1963. *Hallucinogenic Drugs and their Psychotherapeutic Use* (Proceedings of a Meeting of the Association, 1961). London.

SOCIETY FOR PSYCHOSOMATIC RESEARCH. *The Nature of Stress Disorder* (Report of 1958 conference). London.

Index